Feeding the
Body

Nourishing the
Soul

Feeding the
Body
Nourishing the
Soul

ESSENTIALS OF EATING FOR PHYSICAL, EMOTIONAL, AND SPIRITUAL WELL-BEING

DEBORAH KESTEN

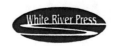

White River Press

FEEDING THE BODY, NOURISHING THE SOUL

Deborah Kesten

Published October 2007 by White River Press
by arrangement with the author

Publication history
Conari Press, copyright 1997

Cover design by Sonja Hakala of White River Press

Interior design by Suzanne Albertson

Grateful acknowledgment is made for permission to reproduce the following: Material adapted with the permission of Rawson Associates/Scribner, an imprint of Simon and Schuster, from *Managing Your Mind and Mood Through Food* by Judith J. Wurtman, Ph.D., Copyright ©1986 Interneuron, Inc., David F. Wurtman and Rachel E. Wurtman. Data for "food-mood guide" taken from *Food: Your Miracle Medicine* by Jean Carper. Copyright ©1993 by Jean Carper. Reprinted by permission of HarperCollins Publishers Inc.

White River Press
PO Box 4624
White River Junction, Vermont 05001
www.whiteriverpress.com

ISBN: 978-0-9792451-3-8

Library of Congress Cataloging-in-Publication Data

Kesten, Deborah, 1948-
  Feeding the body, nourishing the soul : essentials of eating for physical, emotional, and spiritual well-being / Deborah Kesten.
      p. cm.
  Previous ed.: Berkeley, Calif., Conari Press, 1997.
  ISBN 978-0-9792451-3-8 (pbk.)
  1. Food--Religious aspects. 2. Table--Religious aspects. 3. Food--Psychological aspects. 4. Food habits--Psychological aspects. I. Title.
  BL65.F65K47 2007
  613.2--dc22

                        2007030908

This book is dedicated to
my husband Larry,
who brings the smile of
spirituality to all he does.

contents

foreword

Modern nutritional sciences advise us what to eat and what not to eat to maintain health and to help cure our ailments. But the advice often changes and is frequently confusing. Yet there are lasting basic beliefs about food that have been sustained for millennia. In this fascinating and timely book, Deborah Kesten traces the role of food through the wisdom traditions, while reminding us of food's spirituality—an ageless tradition that we may lose by emphasizing only the physically sustaining components of food.

In essence, Deborah Kesten shows us not only how food sustains us by providing bodily fuel, but how it helps to sanctify our lives. Indeed, the association of food with spirituality is a centuries-old, universally accepted concept that is expressed in food-centered ceremonies, rituals, prayers, and holidays that are designed to make food holy. In this way, the age-old propensity to link food with spirituality becomes obvious.

This well-researched and enlightening book explores the spiritual essence of our cultural beliefs surrounding food; as it does, we are given a broad perspective on nutrition—one that integrates mind, body, and spirituality. I have found her message inspiring and worthy of attention.

—Herbert Benson, M.D.
The Mind/Body Medical Institute,
Associate Professor of Medicine,
Harvard Medical School; and
President and Founder of the
Mind/Body Medical Institute, Beth
Israel Deaconess Medical Center,
CareGroup

part one

Food and the
Wisdom Traditions

one

Spirituality: The Missing Ingredient in Food

The truth is that at the end of a well-savored meal
both soul and body enjoy a special well-being ...
the spirit grows more perceptive....[1]

—*Jean Anthelme Brillat-Savarin*

I vividly remember the moment that inspired my search to find the sacred, reverential ingredient in food. I was in New Delhi, India, where I had been invited to give a workshop on "Demystifying Healthful Eating" at the First International Conference on Lifestyle and Health. Many esteemed scientists from throughout India had presented, but one of the most charismatic and intriguing was Hindu cardiologist Dr. K. L. Chopra, father and mentor of the well-known author Deepak Chopra.

After his presentation, I talked with Dr. Chopra in the cavernous auditorium, interviewing him for a magazine article I was planning to write about yoga and diet. When I asked him about his orientation toward food, his response was immediate: "*Prana* is the vital life force of the universe, the cosmic force ... and it goes into you, into me, with food. When you cook with love, you transfer the love into the food and it is metabolized.... In former days (based on the Hindu scripture, the *Bhagavad Gita*), the tradition was for the mother to cook the food with love and then feed it to the children; only then would she eat."

As a nutritionist trained in the scientific method, it seemed incredible to consider that how we think or feel could actually alter food, but Dr. Chopra's comments led me to recall some clues that seemed to fit. For instance, I remembered some close friends telling me that I must have prepared with love a meal they had just eaten; that must be why it was so delicious, they said. I smiled and thanked my friends for their kind words, but inwardly, I wondered at their comment. Around the same time, my husband and I had both noticed on several occasions—independent of each other—that processor-chopped vegetables did not have the same "full" flavor as vegetables we had prepared by hand.

Regardless, I remained skeptical and turned to more rational, familiar explanations: Perhaps because my friends knew that I usually prepared food with care, they anticipated that it would taste good. Perhaps their expectations alone influenced the way they experienced the flavor of the food. Or maybe the food I had made tasted good in its own right.

However, the thought wouldn't let go. Fascinated by the possibility that consciousness could alter the food we eat, I began a search through what philosopher Huston Smith calls the world's "wisdom traditions,"[2] religions and cosmologies that serve as guides for how to live, for their teachings about food. My thinking was that if Hindus believe that loving awareness is somehow transmuted into food—and that we "ingest" this vital force when we eat—then possibly other spiritual traditions would have discovered this too. Inspired by this possibility, I also examined what the biological and behavioral sciences had to say about thoughts, feelings, and food.

As my research intensified, my view of how human beings could best relate to food began to broaden. In the past, I worked diligently to demystify optimal nutrition by researching, writing, counseling, and lecturing about how to follow a low-fat, whole food-based diet. I developed this approach after combining scientific literature reviews on the epidemiology of diet and disease with what I had learned after analyzing scores of diet diaries of patients with heart disease. But now, as I began to study ancient food-related wisdom, my approach expanded to include how our awareness of the sacred—as well as what and how we eat—affects our health.

Although I didn't realize it at the time, my search to find a more integrated approach to eating actually began with traditional nutritional science. For it was within this framework that I had begun my search for the optimal way of eating—the foods that would keep our bodies as healthy as possible. To do this, I majored in the health sciences as an undergraduate, then specialized in public health as a graduate student, obtaining a master's degree in public health.

In graduate school, I began to work as a nutrition educator with Dean Ornish, M.D., author of the bestsellers *Eat More, Weigh Less* and *Dr. Dean Ornish's Program for Reversing Heart Disease.* Dr. Ornish, a medical student at the time, had just finished a pilot study that included treating a small group of heart patients with comprehensive lifestyle changes—a low-fat, vegetarian diet, group support, and stress management.

The project on which I worked as the nutrition educator was the first randomized clinical trial (the "gold standard" of research) to assess the effects of comprehensive lifestyle changes on patients with heart disease. The results of this pioneering research—the first to show that heart health could be significantly improved (fewer angina episodes, improved duration of exercise, lower cholesterol and triglyceride levels, etc.) through the lifestyle changes of a "no-fat-added," plant based diet, exercise, stress management (yoga and meditation), and group support—were published in 1983 in the *Journal of the American Medical Association.*[3]

A decade later, I moved to Europe with my husband, Larry Scherwitz, Ph.D., a behavioral scientist who has worked for many years with Dr. Ornish as co-principal investigator and research director, to learn if this lifestyle program would be relevant in other cultures. For two years, we replicated this lifestyle-change research at cardiovascular rehabilitation clinics in Germany and Holland, and lectured in Germany, England, Sweden, and Switzerland. Our research supported that done in the United States: Consuming fresh, whole, foods—fruits, vegetables, whole grains, legumes (beans and peas), and nonfat dairy products (when combined with other lifestyle approaches) could lower cholesterol and insulin levels, enhance weight loss, decrease depression and anxiety, and even "reverse" blockages in coronary arteries—regardless of one's culture.[4]

But even in the light of such scientific success, I continued to sense that a piece of the nutritional puzzle was missing. I began to wonder where the objective, scientific approach was taking us. Perhaps it was cutting us off from that sense of connection of which Dr. Chopra spoke.

Such sentiments crystallized into an answer one day as I drove up the California coast and pulled into a Chevron station to buy gas. While speaking with the attendant, I learned that Chevron and other gasoline stations were in the process of creating partnerships with McDonald's (called "co-branded on-site locations"[5]) that would make it possible for customers to order fast food while filling the gas tank.

In test sites across the country, customers could scan a menu while at the gas pump, order a hamburger via a speaker or push buttons, and pay with a credit card. Then, as they checked their oil or cleaned their windshield, a McDonald's "crew member" could deliver the food to them. The customers could begin eating the food in their car, while accelerating onto the freeway.

I was stunned about what this and many other "convenience" food trends implied: now we have eating-on-the run; speed is taking precedence over the loving preparation of food; convenience is winning over consciously caring about what's in the food; and a sense of urgency about time is keeping us from savoring the flavor in our food. More and more, we are treating food as merely fuel to keep us going—like gas in a car. Not only are we not paying much attention to how our meals are prepared nor to our state of mind as we eat, we don't even believe these two factors have anything to do with our health or well-being.

I began to wonder if there are consequences for being so disconnected from what we eat, for being so distanced from the connection between ourselves and what and how we eat. Was there really a sacred ingredient—an attitude of appreciation, regard, and reverence—that we could cultivate and bring to the food we eat, as Dr. Chopra's comment implied? Would it make a difference if we approached eating with a more integrated perspective that included not only biological but psychological and sacred awareness?

With these thoughts in mind, I began to perceive that modern nutrition's approach to food is similar to studying the individual threads in a beautiful tapestry in lieu of viewing the whole picture. Analyzing food for its vitamin, mineral, or fat content is comparable to assessing whether the tapestry is made of wool or cotton. Such information could be important, but what's missing is our subjective appreciation of the art itself—its content, the message, and the feelings that the artist is seeking to convey.

By studying the food-related beliefs of various wisdom traditions, I came to regard food as a work of art that needed to be appreciated in its totality. For I discovered that in addition to the Hindu belief that espouses approaching food with loving regard, other wisdom traditions encourage us to honor food, and to partake of it with a depth and sincerity that indeed, make it sacred. I realized that regardless of our personal orientation to food, the wisdom traditions offer a spiritual perspective that somehow we have forgotten over the centuries. The implication: when we furnish food with such sacred understanding, it will nourish both body and soul in ways we have been depriving ourselves of.

To unearth wisdom about the profound meaning of food in our lives, I decided to speak directly with people who had already achieved an enlightened, personal relationship to food. I wanted to capture their unique perspectives about the sacred essence of food as seen through the eyes of their religion, culture, or state-of-the-art research. I wanted their emotional, subjective experience, in addition to what I would research, read about, and study.

With this intention, I interviewed more than forty-five religionists, scientists, and "everyday" people about their food-related beliefs or research. I then assimilated their personal "pearls of wisdom" with my own research and reading about the history and philosophy of these traditions. The first part of this book surveys these traditions one by one. In turn, so that you may derive as much experiential insight as possible, I have included in each chapter a step-by-step description of techniques that can help you create, access, or impart your own sacred ingredients to cooking and eating. Consider applying any or all these practices that call to you in your own kitchen. Only in this way can you discover whether the awareness you bring to food holds the potential both to feed the body and nourish the soul.

As you shall see in these pages, most cultures and religions intuitively have developed rituals that use food as a vehicle to connect to its deeper significance. Judaism's dietary laws are designed to honor the sanctity of life that is in both animal- and plant-based food; Christians honor the divine by connecting to Jesus Christ through the bread and wine of Holy Communion; African Americans celebrate food, life, and friendship by "spicing" soul food with love; yogis eat, in part, to commune with food's life-giving qualities; Muslims honor food for its divine essence; Buddhists pursue enlightenment by bringing a meditative awareness to food; the Chinese use food to communicate with gods; and the Japanese turn to tea to renew the spirit.

In addition to sharing what these spiritual traditions have to tell us about the true nature of our relationship to food, one chapter reveals how transcendence and a sense of connection to nature can be experienced by abstaining from food, as in the Native American fasting tradition of the vision quest. And the chapter on the Hindu wedding feast brings yet another sacred perspective: how sharing a sumptuous, elaborate meal with others can serve as more than a symbol of joyous, sacred fellowship.

Although the wisdom traditions have much to say about the sacred aspect of food, I still remained skeptical about the possibility that human consciousness could actually alter food. To pursue this further, I researched the literature and interviewed scientists, in part to address my own skepticism about the feasibility of imparting loving awareness into the food that we cultivate, prepare, and eat. For if this were possible, then the concept of "nourishment" could be expanded to include not only familiar nutrients, but also sacred sustenance. Would science have something to tell us about such seemingly incredible concepts? I decided to find out.

As I talked with scientists and other pioneers who are examining food and eating in the light of spiritual sustenance, I hoped to see if their research could verify this amazing interconnectedness, this link between consciousness and food. As you will discover, the science and psychologically oriented chapters chart new territory by showing us what happens when we apply the scientific method to the "new" nutrition paradigm that ancient cultures and religions have sensed intuitively over the centuries.

I first write about the psychological connection in Chapter 12, "The Starving Spirit," which addresses my hypothesis that eating disorders—anorexia, bulimia, and overeating—emerge when the link between food and spirit is severed. My thesis: If the wisdom traditions espouse that we bring a loving, sacred awareness to our food, then perhaps the converse of this relationship—lack of love (a "starving spirit")—is related to eating disorders.

I wrote the next chapter, "The Food-Mood Connection," to examine the effects food has on our emotions, while "Spiritually Imbued Food" shows exactly what science had to say about food that has been intentionally imbued with loving, conscious energy. This chapter attempts to answer the question that inspired this book: Does bringing a loving awareness to food really affect it? Finally, "Food Meditation: Creating Conscious Connection," shows you even more in-depth how to apply and use the food-related wisdom of both the ancient traditions and science, so that you may create your own sacred connection to food.

As you journey through the various "spiritual kitchens" and scientific laboratories in this book, it is my hope that you will sense the potential grandeur of your sacred relationship to food. Along the way, may you discover your own recipes to nourish both body and soul.

two

Judaism: Divine Dietary Tradition

Jewish dietary laws reflect—and mirror... a more-or-less true understanding... of the nature and the place of man within the whole.... They... pay homage to... the dignity of life.... These remarkable customs not only restrain and thwart the bad, they also commemorate the true and beckon... us toward holiness.[1]

—*Leon R. Kass, M.D.*

Steeped in centuries of tradition, Judaism has always held a profound reverence and compassion for all life. Given this heritage—more likely, **because** of this essential value—for more than 3,000 years devout Jews have turned to dialogue, debate, and dialectics to define the "eating style" that most accurately reflects Jewish concepts of holiness: the pure plant-based diet of Adam and Eve, a meat-inclusive diet, and the dietary rules of *Kashrut* that define ritually pure, kosher food. Regardless of where they are on the dietary spectrum, all practicing Jews have in common a belief in the humane heritage of Jewish tradition. On one level, such philosophical issues about Judaism's dietary laws challenge mind and soul, asking us to pay attention to the foods we choose in our everyday life. On a more profound level, Judaism's dietary laws inspire us to value them as a "golden thread" that links the food we eat to the compassionate core of this ancient faith.

Sabbath Savories and Sentiments

A delicious aroma fills Richard Schwartz' home. It is just before sunset on Friday evening, and the glow of the Sabbath (from the Hebrew word *Shabbat*, meaning "rest") fills his heart and that of his family: his wife, Loretta, three grown children, two sons-in-law, and five grandchildren. Standing, Loretta lights the Sabbath candles while reciting a blessing over them: *Blessed art Thou, O Lord our God, Creator of the Universe, Who has made us holy by Thy Laws and commanded us to light the Sabbath lights.*

Then, after Friday evening services, the family sings songs that welcome the Sabbath angels of peace. Afterward, resting both of his hands on the heads of each child and grandchild present, Schwartz blesses them in turn with the traditional Jewish blessing that seeks God's benevolence, protection, and graciousness.

Next, with the family in a joyous mood, Schwartz picks up the *Kiddush* cup, the special cup that holds the Sabbath wine, or grape juice, that symbolizes holiness and joy and a brimful of blessings. With the Kiddush cup raised, he chants the special blessing: *Blessed art Thou, O Lord our God, Creator of the Universe, Who creates the fruit of the vine.* Then he drinks from this "cup of joy," recalling his choice to choose good over evil. As he does so, the Sabbath is made holy.[2]

After a symbolic washing of hands, Schwartz then recites a blessing over the *challah*, a loaf of "braided" bread that symbolizes the years the Israelites spent in the wilderness on their way to the Promised Land. The two loaves of challah on the table represent the double portions of manna (a breadlike substance) the ancient Israelites gathered on Friday, so they would not have to go out and gather manna on Saturday, the Sabbath day. Each member of the family then eats a bit of the challah as Schwartz says a blessing: *Blessed art Thou, O Lord our God, Creator of the Universe, Who brings forth bread from the earth.* Now, along with songs that thank God for this day of rest, and for home and family, everyone partakes in the good food on the table. *Shabbat Shalom,* everyone says: "Peace to you on the Sabbath."

For the Schwartz family, the Sabbath food is vegetarian—mostly fruits, vegetables, grains, legumes, nuts, and seeds. On this particular Sabbath evening, dinner includes a potpourri of meatless dishes, ranging from mushroom-barley soup and green salad to potato kugel, rice pilaf, a vegetable casserole, and other side dishes such as corn and a cranberry-applesauce mixture.

The next morning, the Schwartz family participates in religious services at the synagogue. "After the service," explains Richard, "we return home to another traditional Jewish vegetarian meal." However, this time when he chants the *Kiddush* with wine, it includes the Biblical verse that indicates that animals as well as people are to rest on the Sabbath day.

Similar sentiments of appreciation are present when he says prayers over the two loaves of challah. "I often think of the miraculous processes that have brought this food to our table—from the planting of the seeds to the final product. Then we have the meal, which includes all kinds of vegetarian foods. In the winter months, this may include *cholent*, a Yiddish word that describes a casserole of potatoes, carrots, all kinds of beans, and seasonings, which we cook slowly in a crockpot for many hours before and during the Sabbath." (Lights, including flames from the stove, can neither be turned on nor kindled during the Sabbath.)

Toward dusk, after a day of resting, thinking, reading, or playing (just *being* rather than *doing*), and a prescribed "third meal," the Sabbath ends when three stars can be seen in the sky. This transition—between the Sabbath and the other days of the week—is also celebrated with blessings. Called *Havdalah*, meaning "separation," the informal farewell calls for a wine cup, a candle, and a box filled with spices.

May the coming week overflow with goodness like the wine in the cup,[3] says Richard, holding the *Kiddush* cup as it brims with wine. Then he lights a special candle made of twisted strands that symbolize the many different kinds of light God created—the light of the sun, moon, and stars—and the Jewish laws by which to live. During the *Havdalah*, Schwartz opens a spice box (a replacement for the incense-burning of ancient times), releasing the fragrant scent of cloves, nutmeg, and bay leaves. The symbolism: hope for a week that will be pleasant and "sweet-smelling."

Now the sun has set and the Sabbath is over—until next Friday at sunset.

Divine Dietary Consciousness

Richard Schwartz and his family are celebrating the Jewish Sabbath, an ancient, holy, twenty-four-hour period that has been celebrated by Jews since Biblical times. On this special day, the finest meals of the week are served. For most Jews, along with the twisted challah bread, the meal consists of fish, fowl, or meat with side dishes of various vegetables. Some families drink wine; others choose grape juice to represent the joy of the Sabbath.

Regardless of the specific dishes served in each family, the selected foods—and their preparation—are based on a tradition of Biblical dietary laws (*Kashrut* in Hebrew). While observant Jews follow the laws of *Kashrut* because they believe it is God's will, perhaps understanding the moral compassion at the core of Judaism's dietary laws reveals the wisdom of how to "be" in the world regardless of religion.

Says philosopher and author Leon R. Kass, M.D., in *The Hungry Soul: Eating and the Perfecting of Our Nature*, "[Judaism's dietary laws] manifest a more or less true understanding of the world, including the place of man within the whole."[4] At their core, the dietary laws are designed to inspire a sense of oneness and connection to God, giving the Jewish people an opportunity to express their holiness at every meal.[5]

Indeed, when interpreted from the heart, the dietary laws become meaningful guidelines by which to live, rather than a list of seemingly antiquated and literal dietary "do's and don'ts." Says Rabbi Harold Schulweis of Temple Valley Beth Shalom in Encino, California, "The Jewish belief is that when you take food, you dedicate it toward that which rejoices the heart. This is done through *prayer,* which means 'the sacrifice of the heart, the work of the heart.'"

Rabbi Schulweis bases his beliefs on "a part of the Jewish tradition that," he says, "has been buried, repressed, not spoken of." I spoke with Rabbi Schulweis in his office during a visit to his synagogue in Southern California.[6] "Many of us have forgotten the teleology," he says, "the purpose and rationale behind Jewish dietary laws."

By remembering the underlying purpose of *Kashrut,* Richard Schwartz believes we may reconnect with their original holy intent. For dietary observances, important though they are in the scheme of Judaism, are meaningful only in the context of God's covenant with the ancient Israelites—an "agreement" that showing compassion, reverence, and appreciation for nature's bounty and all life, including animals, is to be Godlike.

The Past in the Present

The Jewish tradition of keeping *kosher*—eating certain foods prepared in a particular way—has roots in both the Hebrew Bible (the *Pentateuch:* the first five books of Moses, the *Words of the Prophets,* and other sacred writings, including psalms and proverbs), and the *Talmud* (ancient oral teachings and discussions of Biblical concepts by rabbis, teachers of the Jewish religion). Reinterpreted over time by generations of rabbis, these traditional laws have evolved into the dietary laws that many Jews follow today.

To understand the essence of the dietary laws is to realize that Judaism is not wholly a religion of dogma. Indeed, one of its distinguishing features is a love of learning, especially interpretations of the written and oral *Torah,* the Hebrew word for *teaching* or *law,* by which Jews live. This is manifested through various interpretations of the laws over time.

For instance, Orthodox Judaism holds fast to uncompromising observance of the dietary laws in the *Pentateuch,* as interpreted by Talmudic sages, because they are considered to be the words of God;

Orthodox Hasidic Jews have adopted even more stringent dietary laws than those observed by Orthodox Jews.[7] The more liberal Reform Judaism encourages its adherents to interpret the dietary laws according to their own conscience and moral values, rather than the written word; and "middle-of-the-road" Conservative Judaism considers the dietary laws to have "evolved through the historical experience of the Jewish people.... They are therefore (perceived to be) part of the divine-human encounter (that) can serve in the present ... in *furthering the ideal of holiness in daily living.*"[8]

In addition to the traditional interpretations of the dietary laws by various denominations, a small but growing number of Orthodox, Reform, and Conservative rabbis, theologians, and practitioners have interpreted Judaism's dietary laws (and other Jewish values and teachings) as a call to vegetarianism. They believe that to respect the sanctity of all life and show compassion is to eschew flesh and eat a plant-based diet—as do Richard Schwartz and his family. Comments Rabbi Schulweis, who defines himself as a "fishaterian": "It seems to me that the basic, spiritual, underlying concern in Judaism is the sanctity of life.... If you are having this treaty with nature, this harmony ... it would be a logical extension to see to it that the meal is without the death of an animal."

Regardless of how God's dietary laws are interpreted—literally, metaphorically, morally, or ethically—each denomination shares a common tenet: that all food should be savored with a sense of holiness. In other words, whether or not meat is included in a meal, Judaism regards food as sacred, an opportunity to connect with God. Writes anthropologist Mary Douglas in *Purity and Danger:* "the dietary laws ... have been like signs which at every turn inspired meditation on the oneness, purity, and completeness of God."[9]

Evolving Dietary Rules

The sense of sacredness linked to Judaism's current dietary laws is expressed throughout their evolution in the *Torah* from Adam and Eve to Noah to God's Biblical *Kashrut.* Interestingly, each stage is related to what is *forbidden*—from eating the apple from the tree of knowledge, to the consumption of blood (seen as the life force in an animal), to various kinds of animals, fish, and fowl. Many theologians and philosophers speculate that such laws are God's way of curtailing humankind's propensity for out-of-control excess and gluttony in all aspects of living—including what, when, and how we eat. Rabbi Schulweis uses the term "refined consciousness" to express the awareness and appreciation the dietary laws ask Jews to bring to food, especially animal-based food.

The first reference to food (and human issues surrounding it) occurs in the Garden of Eden where Adam and Eve lived on a plant-based diet. The first creation story in the *Torah* presents the paradise that is Eden as a land filled with "seed-bearing plants which are on the face of all the earth, and every tree which has seed-bearing fruit; to you I have given it as food." (Genesis 1:29–30).

This idyll was not to last. For after Eve eats the apple from the forbidden tree of knowledge, she and Adam are no longer innocent children of God; they have now discovered free choice and, therefore, the potential for excess and "being human." Finally expelled from the garden, Adam and Eve's descendants turn from fruit to the cultivation of grain and the making of bread.

As civilization grows, the *Torah* tells us, so too does humankind's propensity for meat. The most prevailing motive appears to be the human being's pure enjoyment of meat. Writes Rabbi Schulweis: "God discovers that the human being has powerful, instinctive drives … loves meat rare or well done."[10] Indeed, in a world of animal sacrifice and ritual, hot weather, and no refrigeration with which to keep meat fresh, Rabbi Schulweis explained, it was not unusual for pagans to consume animal meat and parts without regard to the welfare of the animal.

Conceding to these seemingly inherent desires and violent tendencies, God gives Noah and his descendants (and therefore, all humans) permission to be carnivorous—but with one qualification:

the consumption of blood was forbidden. Writes Rabbi Edward Rosenthal in the chapter he contributed to *Rabbis and Vegetarianism:* "The Torah allows them [human beings] to vent their passions and assert dominion over all those creatures for whom they previously served as caretakers and protectors," yet "to remove the blood is the minimum requirement of humane treatment"[11] required of both Jews and the rest of humanity.

Refined Consciousness

These Noahic food practices continued for centuries, but after the Temple in Jerusalem was destroyed, rabbis, interpreting the *Torah*, replaced the consumption of meat, connected with animal sacrifices, with what has come to be called the dietary laws of *Kashrut*. By commanding that the Jewish people "should not be given a free rein to slaughter and eat anything that walks, crawls, slithers, hops, flies, or swims . . . (this brought) an awareness of and consideration for the life which is taken to create food,"[12] writes Rabbi Rosenthal. In essence, these laws raised "that which was considered to be ordinary and profane to a level of holiness."

After the destruction of the Temple, another major change occurred between Jews and their relationship to food. No longer able to practice animal sacrifice in the temple, "study and prayer took the place of sacrifice," explains Rabbi Schulweis, "and so study itself became holy." The word for *prayer*—and study if it is part of prayer—means "the sacrifice of the heart, the work of the heart. After the deluge, food and meals were accompanied with prayer, the work of the heart."

By bringing a prayerful consciousness to food and an awareness of the life that was taken to create the food, these dietary laws became more than commandments to be followed. For underlying the what-to-eat, what-not-to-eat rules is an intricately worked tapestry that weaves together human values and ethical sensibilities with the type of animal-based foods that are consumed. In essence, writes Max

Friedman, the dietary laws "served as a reminder that the animal being eaten is a creature of God, [and] that the death of such a creature cannot be taken lightly."[13] Explains Rabbi Schulweis: "God is saying, If you must eat meat, do so with awareness that you are taking the life of another. If you must take the life of another, see to it that it is done with compassion."[14]

Other Jewish theologians speculate that God created dietary dictums to enhance the holiness of the Jews, minimizing what author Mary Douglas refers to as "secular defilement."[15] For they also served as a symbol of holiness, preserving the monotheism of God's people, and setting them apart from surrounding pagan societies who continued to ravage animals indiscriminately.

But perhaps, as a contrast to pagan sensibilities, the dietary laws also created a more refined, more meaningful, Godlike way in which the Jewish people could connect to food. Says Rabbi Schulweis: "The Biblical dietary laws sensitized people...made them more *refined* [emphasis added]. Jews no longer looked at the environment of animals, and anything taken from them, without awareness." Adds Dr. Leon Kass: "The laws intend to provide a discipline good for the soul, partly by the mere acts of self-denial of particular animal foods, but mainly by the need to attend scrupulously to details of the diet."[16]

What exactly are these "dietary details"? On an objective level, they are mostly a conglomeration of Biblical statutes and rabbinic interpretation and legislation that have evolved over the centuries. But behind the words lie a deeper meaning and purpose that a growing number of Jewish scholars and theologians have been exploring. Specifically, they are "rediscovering" the moral intent and holiness inherent in these laws. For many of the forbidden foods (all of which are animal-based) are either literally or metaphorically related to an animal's or human being's degree of aggression or "refined consciousness."

Setting the Kosher Table

Plant-based food. In essence, writes Richard Schwartz, Ph.D., in his book, *Judaism and Vegetarianism:* "God's first dietary law...is a spiritual blueprint of a vegetarian world order."[17] The Bible tells us that much of the food consumed by Israelites in the Holy Land consisted of fruits, vegetables, grains, legumes, nuts, and seeds. Common fruits included figs, pomegranates, dates, olives and their oil, and grapes that were made into wine.[18] Typical vegetables included wild vegetables, leeks, squash, cucumbers, and onions. Corn was especially popular, as was cracked wheat (bulgar) barley, and spelt, another type of grain. Grains were either roasted or ground for use in baked goods, such as bread. Because *unleavened* bread (yeast-free) was seen as a gift from *Yahweh* (the ancient Hebrews' word for God), it was considered holy; adding yeast, therefore, was seen as disrespectful and profane.[19] A limited amount of legumes were available; lentils were typical Biblical fare. Pistachios, almonds, and sesame seeds were typical nuts and seeds included in the diet.

Dairy. The ancient Israelites depended on milk and its products, from sheep or goats, as a staple, nourishing food. But because pagans would cook a young goat in its mother's milk, the Bible forbade Jews to continue this practice, perceiving it as symbolically cruel and inhumane. Although the original law applied only to mixing milk and its products with animals sacrificed at the altar (especially a lamb), the *Talmud* expanded this concept to include all animals and fowl. Specifically, milk and its products, such as butter, cheese, and cream, may not be eaten or cooked together with meat, or used for monetary profit.[20] This included not eating dairy-containing dishes such as desserts with meat dishes. To honor this moral concept and ensure the separation of milk and meat, rabbis introduced separate sets of dishes and utensils into the kosher home.

Meat, poultry, fish. In order to ensure regard for the sanctity of animals slaughtered for food, the ancient kosher laws specified certain *permitted* animals, as well as the specific *method* by which they should be killed. While hygienic considerations may have played a role in the evolution of the laws, this was not their only purpose. As previously mentioned, they also served as a symbolic expression of Jews' love for and relationship with God via a conscious reverence and compassion for the life God had given to animals.

Mostly, though, the rules regarding meat focus on forbidden and permitted animals, fowl, and fish. For instance, acceptable animals (considered "clean") include those with cloven hooves that consume plant-based foods by chewing the cud (sheep, goats, and cattle), but not swine, hares, or camels; fish with fins and scales (trout, salmon, flounder), but not shellfish (shrimp, lobster, clams); and nonanimal-eating birds, such as chicken, turkey, and duck, but not, for instance, eagles, owls, and ravens; certain winged insects are also forbidden.

Eggs, too, are part of the kosher diet. They are used as daily dietary fare, but are also part of many joyous holidays such as Passover when a hard-boiled egg, believed to signify rebirth, is included in the ritual.

In addition, because blood symbolized God-given life, it continued to be forbidden. Any remaining blood from a slaughtered animal was to be drawn off by presoaking and salting the meat.

Compassionate slaughter. Kosher dietary laws passed down over the centuries by rabbis further refined and defined kosher food and acceptable and unacceptable behavior surrounding its preparation. After the Jews were exiled from Palestine in the first century CE, the compassionate, ritualistic slaughter of animals became mandatory in order to minimize any animal's suffering. The ritualistic slaughtering is based on Judaism's abhorrence of taking life, and its commitment to compassion for animals. Says Rabbi Schulweis: "The very first law of *Kashrut* is: You cannot eat a limb from a living creature. This initiated laws about the ritual slaughter of animals *(shechitah)* that is subject to specific, very detailed laws. For instance, a *shochet* (a person specially trained to slaughter animals for food) must use a special notch-free knife, and withdraw it quickly, without any hesitation or delay."

As a matter of fact, out of respect for the welfare of an animal, before saying grace and after a meal, today's devout Jews are asked to remove knives from the table. "There's something contradictory about pleasing God, producing food, and then having the instrument that is used to kill, cut, and maim rest on the table," explains Rabbi Schulweis. "This custom is no longer followed, but I believe it has to be revived."

To illustrate how the moral values are woven into the customs of the Jewish people, Rabbi Schulweis, in his chapter in *Rabbis and Vegetarianism,* tells this rabbinic anecdote about a new *shochet* "who was to replace the beloved old *shochet* who had passed. They tested the new *shochet* and someone asked, 'How did he do?' One of the men sighed.

> 'What's the matter? Didn't he recite the prayers?'
> 'He did.'
> 'Didn't he sharpen the knife?'
> 'He did.'
> 'Didn't he moisten the blade?'
> 'He did.'
> 'What was wrong then?
> 'Well,' the man said, 'our old *shochet* used to moisten the blade with his tears.'"[21]

There are additional behavioral refinements based on Judaism's holy dietary laws. "If you're going to take the eggs from a mother hen, you must first chase the hen away, because it is considered cruel for the mother to see her eggs taken away," explains Rabbi Schulweis. Hunting, too, is not considered kosher. "The idea of shooting down an animal just for fun … is a profoundly un-Jewish activity," he says.

Rules with Reason

Anthropologist Mary Douglas also believes that the dietary laws surrounding animal-based food serve as a reminder to Jews of the purity and perfection that is God. Seen with this insight, every meal becomes a connection to holiness, an opportunity to connect with God, she says.[22]

Dr. Leon Kass agrees that "the true concern of the dietary laws is holiness." Indeed, he attributes an intricate web of both rational and spiritual meaning to the animal-related rules. Specifically, he prescribes much significance to the *place, form, motion,* and *life* of various animals.

In his book *The Hungry Soul: Eating and the Perfecting of Our Nature,* Dr. Kass correlates the dietary rules to the *places* inhabited by animals: land, water, and air. He writes: "I observe that the criteria used to identify the clean and the unclean [animals] refer to their *form,* their *means of motion,* and how they *sustain* life—that is, what they eat to live—specifically, whether they eat other animals or not."

In other words, by considering animals, fish, fowl, and insects in regard to their relationship to the whole of how they are in the world, we are given a perspective as to whether they "least disturb the created order." In essence, the Children of Israel are asked "not to incorporate animals that kill and incorporate other animals," says Dr. Kass. By doing so, we are reminded "not only of the created *order* but of the order as *created.*" In turn, "mindful eaters [are reminded] of the supreme rule of the Holy One" and the wisdom of the dietary rules.

Writing in *The Hungry Soul,* Dr. Kass says that "in a certain sense the dietary laws push the Children of Israel back in the direction of the 'original vegetarianism' of the . . . Garden of Eden." His rationale? "Although not all flesh is forbidden, everything that is forbidden is flesh." Thus any strict vegetarian never violates the Jewish dietary laws. "Yet why," he asks, "does not the *Torah* institute other dietary laws that push back all the way to vegetarianism, reversing altogether the Noahic permission to eat meat? Is not vegetarianism the Biblical ideal?"[23]

Professor Richard Schwartz, along with a small but growing number of Jews, argues that vegetarianism is, indeed, the Biblical ideal. Schwartz' odyssey into Judaism and vegetarianism began in the mid-seventies while teaching mathematics and the environment at The College of Staten Island. The purpose of his course was to motivate students by applying basic mathematical concepts to "real life" issues. Their first issue: the crosscultural problem of world hunger.

While doing research, Schwartz realized that 70 percent of the grain produced in the United States was being fed to "food" animals. After sharing this with his students, he gave up red meat and, soon after that, other animal-based foods. "Since then, vegetarianism and its relationship to Judaism has become a dominant part of my life," he told me during a phone conversation between one of his trips to Israel, where he lectures and has initiated the "Campaign for a Vegetarian-Conscious Israel by the Year 2000."

Schwartz stresses six *Torah*-based guideposts that merge what he refers to as "the spirit of Jewish values" with a vegetarian consciousness. "Fortunately, we do not have an either/or situation," he says. "Jewish vegetarians are not placing so-called vegetarian values above *Torah* principles. Rather, they are stressing that basic Jewish teachings mandate treating animals with compassion; guarding our health (by avoiding high-fat, high-cholesterol animal foods); sharing with hungry people; protecting the environment; conserving resources; and seeking peace."[24]

Creating a "Kosher Consciousness"

For more than thirty-odd centuries, one way in which Judaism has "attended" to moral and ethical issues is by highlighting the consciousness surrounding food. In its wisdom, Judaism has created a tradition of discussion and debate, leaving room for interpretation of dietary and other Talmudic laws. For some, this may mean following the dietary laws as God's given word; others may choose to resonate with the "kosher consciousness" by following a vegetarian diet advocated by Schwartz and others.

At its core, the Judaic tradition tells us that food is life entering the body and sustaining it; that it is a "medium" between God and humankind; that it is a connection with both God and our own

Godliness. Because of this, our relationship to food is seen as holy.

Writer Henri Daniel-Rops tells us that the early Israelites considered food to be sacred, and that they acknowledged the hand of God in their daily food by saying a prayer over it and all else that God had provided. The intention of prayer was to "raise a man above himself ... and bring him into a loving relationship with God and generally cause his soul to overcome all that is earthly and material," while remembering that food and other "earthly and material aspects of life had been blessed by God."[25]

Eating "From the Heart"

No matter our spiritual orientation, each time we eat, we have an opportunity to enter into a "prayerful consciousness" and experience Judaism's divine dietary wisdom. What follows are Rabbi Schulweis' suggestions for bringing a Kosher consciousness to each meal, and in the process, do what he refers to as "the work of the heart."

Bless the bread. "A blessing is where heaven and earth, God and the human being, meet; blessing food is a transaction between the food that is given by God and the work of the hands of a human being. Recite the *moszi,* the blessing, over baked bread: *Blessed art Thou who brings forth the bread from the earth.* Keep in mind that breaking bread is the first contact that one has with the meal: the seed, the sun, the soil, the water are given to us by God, but for them to be blessed, one has to plow the soil, nurture the earth, reap the harvest, grind the wheat, mix the four, and make it edible for human beings."

Sanctify wine. "The *Kiddush* is *not* a blessing over grapes; rather, it is over that which has been squeezed, fermented, and prepared by human wisdom and purpose. It is also a union between God and humankind. It says: *Blessed art Thou, O Lord our God, Creator of the Universe, Who creates the fruit of the vine.* The Jewish tradition sublimates the ability of wine to intoxicate by dedicating the wine to spiritual ends, i.e., rejoicing the heart of humankind. For instance, the meal at which wine is served should include the hungry, a stranger. In this sense, wine can take on a different meaning, because it rejoices the heart of the hungry."

Feed the hungry. "Judaism believes that joy is sanctified when it is attached to a moral purpose. In this light, it integrates the material and spiritual worlds by being concerned with the spirit without neglecting the material needs of human beings. This can be seen in the aphorism of the rabbis who say if there is no bread, there is no *Torah* (the body of Jewish literature); if there is no *Torah*, there is no bread. This means that people cannot pray and develop spiritually on an empty stomach. Therefore, before preaching spiritually to the hungry, feed them."

Bring sacred awareness to each meal. "The Hebrew Bible is a sublime liturgy of thanksgiving to God, acknowledging the Creator's hand in the gift of food and drink. Because such nourishment is part of the divine plan, the Bible tells us to honor eating and drinking as hallowed activities. Judaism also posits that both the liturgy and prayers tell us that the body and soul are one. Therefore, drink and food are not disassociated from the spirit. For the spirit cannot live without the body, and the body cannot manifest fully without the spirit. Therein lies the sacredness of the meal."

three

Christianity: The Sacred Supper

Holy God, as you feed me
Spiritually with the Eucharist
Remind me of the great sacrifice
And the love of Jesus.[1]

—Father Robert Bryant,
Episcopal priest

Because there is one bread, we who are many are
one body, for we all partake of the one loaf.[2]

—1 Corinthians 10:16–17

The miracle of the loaves and fishes, when Jesus of Nazareth multiplied five loaves of bread and two fish in order to feed 5,000 people; the wedding banquet wherein Jesus transformed water into wine; the bounty of fish that manifested after Jesus admonished fishermen to cast their nets on the other side of their boat—the **New Testament** is resplendent with food miracles that show us how to be nourished with God's divine grace. But it is the liturgy of the **Last Supper** (also called the Eucharist, Divine Liturgy, Holy Communion, Meal, or the Lord's Supper) that is a food miracle in a realm of its own. As the heart and soul for many of the Christian faith, it transforms either literally or symbolically (depending on the denomination) Jesus' body and blood into **bread** and **wine.** As the essence of Christianity's divine faith, hope, and love, participating in the Eucharist (from the Greek word **Eucharisto,** meaning "to give thanks") provides spiritual nourishment that a community of believers are invited to savor and ingest each time they participate in the Sacred Supper and the mystery of this holy union.

Sharing the Eucharistic Table

Outside the massive Gothic-style grand cathedral in Barcelona, Spain, the sun is hot and glaring. Inside the church, with its massive arches and vast high spaces, it is gray and cool—except for the warmth radiating from the white votive candles that are flickering near the altar. Resting on the altar is a tabernacle, a holy receptacle that holds bread, which has been consecrated into the presence of Jesus Christ through prayers said by the Catholic priest.

American traveler Arthur Manetta has entered the church to participate in the celebration of the *Eucharist*, the Christian sacrament that commemorates Christ's Last Supper. After seating himself on a worn, hand-carved wooden pew, he, along with other members of the congregation, participate in prayers, hymns, and reading scripture. Surrounded by the glow of a special light that seems to radiate throughout the church, he is absorbed by the ethereal sounds of people singing hymns accompanied by an organist and praying in Catalan (an inherently melodious language with which he is unfamiliar). His senses are absorbed by the beauty: diffused lighting, melodious music from the congregation, the scent of burning candles and incense, the general drama and majesty of the Mass, and the grandiosity of the cathedral itself.

Before the priest begins the *offertory*—the offering of bread and wine to God—people in the congregation greet each other with smiles or handshakes, while remaining at their pews. There is a sense of humility, of ordinariness, a solidarity. Then Manetta watches silently as the priest places some hosts (small, round, thin pieces of unleavened bread) onto a paten (the plate that holds the Eucharistic bread), then pours a small portion of wine into a gold chalice. Next, lifting the bread, the priest continues the divine liturgy by consecrating the bread and wine on behalf of the Catholic church.

The priest takes the bread and raises it while saying:
> *For in the night in which he was betrayed, he took bread; and when he had given thanks, he broke it, and gave it to his disciples, saying,*

"Take, eat, this is my body, which is given for you. Do this in remembrance of me."

After raising the chalice that holds the wine, the priest genuflects:
Likewise, after supper, he took the cup; and when he had given thanks, he gave it to them, saying, "Drink ye all of this; for this is my Blood of the New Testament, which is shed for you, and for many, for the remission of sins. Do this, as oft as ye shall drink it, in remembrance of me."

In unison, the participants say "Amen." Now that the bread and wine have been consecrated by the priest (the agent of the Catholic Church), they *are* the body and blood of Christ—although their outward appearance seems unchanged; the transubstantiation is complete.

The Lord's Prayer, the pinnacle of the service, follows. It may be recited, sung, or chanted; regardless of the form in which it is expressed, it is always an integral part of the Mass:

Our Father in heaven,
Hallowed be your name,
Your kingdom come,
Your will be done,
On earth as in heaven.
Give us today our daily bread.... [Amen.]

To signal that the Communion is at hand, an usher appears at the pews, and "the congregation's attention turns to greet Christ in the Eucharist," says author Kevin Orlin Johnson, Ph.D.[3] For those who wish to participate in the taking of the Eucharist, the usher is available to direct them from their benches toward the altar, where the priest stands before the Holy Table.

Walking up the aisle with the other participants, Manetta notes the multitude of statues throughout the church. As an architect, he knows that the statues and richly colored stained-glass windows originally were created to tell the Christian story to preliterate populations, many of whom were uneducated, with limited language skills and different dialects.

Then the priest distributes small portions of the blessed bread by presenting a piece to each of the communicants. When it is Manetta's turn to approach the holy table, the priest places the small piece of bread (the host) in Arthur's mouth, saying: "The body of Christ"; Manetta responds: "Amen." (In many churches, the priest and Eucharistic ministers of men and women often place the bread in the communicants' hands.)

Moments of silent prayer and reflection follow, until the priest marks the end of the Mass with a blessing. Spiritually renewed, Manetta and the other participants rise and walk through the ancient church's portal out into the bright light of day.

Savoring the Savior

For more than forty years, Arthur Manetta has been participating in the observance that is the Eucharist. Baptized a Catholic in his infancy, as an adult he chose to express his spiritual relationship to Christianity and the Eucharistic holy observance by becoming an Episcopalian, one of the Protestant denominations of Christianity.

Regardless of the denomination—Catholic or Protestant—the taking of the bread and wine of the Eucharist has a relevance to something much larger than the ritual itself. For by inviting Christians to experience Jesus' Godliness through the ingestion of the bread and wine, the Eucharist feeds multidimensional hunger. "It is not by any casual coincidence that the presence and saving power of Jesus is set forth in the Eucharist in the form of food," writes Monika K. Hellwig, Ph.D., "because it is a response to hunger...at many levels."[4]

Indeed, reflecting upon his Eucharistic experience in the Gothic cathedral in Barcelona, Manetta told me that he finds participation in the Eucharist to be physically, emotionally, and spiritually fulfilling: "I received multiple levels of nourishment in the cathedral in Barcelona. On the most basic level, there's the *physical* nourishment of the bread and wine; *emotionally* I feel loved and part of something, because God chose to become ordinary so that He could provide a message of

Godliness to us; and I'm nourished *spiritually* because Jesus' Godliness is a manifestation of God in human terms. As important is the connection of sharing a spiritual moment with others."[5]

When interpreted as sustenance for body, mind, heart, and soul, participating in the Eucharist becomes an opportunity to commune with God, and God in the communion of man — rather than mere participation in an ancient ritual. "Yet different Christian traditions offer different Eucharistic experiences," says Father Robert Bryant of the Episcopal Church of Our Saviour in Mill Valley, California.[6] For instance, "Roman Catholics, Orthodox Christians, and Anglicans believe that in the blessing of the bread, Christ becomes truly present; this is the essence of the Roman Catholic doctrine of transubstantiation," which attempts to define the meaning of the taking of the Eucharist.

"Episcopal or Anglican understanding is essentially the same as the Roman Catholic understanding," continues Father Bryant. These denominations believe "that the bread and wine *are* the body of Christ. However, almost all Protestant churches (Baptists, Methodists, etc.) see the Eucharist as a memorial meal," he says, "something that is done to *remember* Jesus' sacrifice." And Quakers are an example of one of a few Christian denominations that do not celebrate the Eucharist at all.

Essentially, one denomination may see the taking of the Eucharist as a literal fulfillment of the words and promise of Jesus, while others interpret it symbolically. The reasons for different interpretations lie in the history of the various Christian churches and the evolution of their various theologies over the centuries.

Participating in the Past

Regardless of their interpretation of the Eucharist, most Christians would agree that it is a repository of God-filled wisdom that encourages spiritual sustenance through the "taking in" of Jesus' Godliness and presence, and doing so while in communion with others. Says writer Hughes Oliphant Old: "Participating in the sacred meal seals the covenantal union between us and our God. Not only does the sacrament bring us into communion with God, it brings us into the Christian community."[7] In addition, says Father Bryant, "the Eucharist tells us that neither life nor death can separate us from the love of God, which is ours in Christ Jesus. For the Eucharist is entering the reality of Christ sacrificed, his death and resurrection."

This participation began two thousand years ago during Jesus' Last Supper, the farewell Passover meal Jesus held with his disciples before his crucifixion. On this night, during what most theologians believe was a celebration of the Jewish Passover (Seder) meal, Jesus selected unleavened bread and wine, blessed the bread and wine, gave thanks, then broke the bread and poured the wine while telling his disciples: "This is my body, broken for you," and "This is my blood, the blood of the covenant, which is to be poured out for many."[8] The Gospel according to John, which most scholars believe includes John's reflections on the origins of the mystery of the Eucharist, tells us that Jesus said:

> *"I am the bread of life; he who comes to me shall not hunger, and he who believes in me shall never thirst... He who eats my flesh and drinks my blood abides in me, and I in him. As the living Father sent me, and I live because of the Father, so he who eats of me will live because of me."*[9]

After distributing the pieces of bread and wine to his disciples, Jesus told them to repeat the breaking of bread and the drinking of wine after his death to signify their taking communion with him via his death and resurrection. Said Jesus: "For as often as you eat the bread and drink the cup, you proclaim the Lord's death until he comes."[10] And with these words and the offering of his body and blood—his very life—for others through the taking of the bread and wine, the sacrament of Holy Communion was born.

In the early days after Jesus' crucifixion, local followers took part in the Eucharist in the privacy of their own homes. Gathering in

Jesus' name, they integrated the breaking of bread and drinking of wine into their ordinary meals. For these early Christians, the sharing of both a meal and the Eucharist added to their sense of purpose.[11] For Jesus had ministered while dining not only with his disciples, but with a motley assortment of others, ranging from prostitutes to beggars. So, too, when early Christians sat down to share a meal, it embodied a spiritual occasion that expressed equality with others in the eyes of God.

"The sharing of food had more significance at that time than it does now," says Clayton Harrop, Ph.D., Senior Professor of New Testament at Golden Gate Baptist Theological Seminary.[12] I spoke with Dr. Harrop in his office at the Baptist institution in Mill Valley, California. "Jesus' teachings tell us that every believer has a right to gather around the table and share a meal. In other words, there are no distinctions of any kind among Christians. Whatever your background, whether rich or poor, regardless of the clothes you wear, your racial heritage, or past deeds, we are all one in our relationship with God.

"In Paul's writings [one of Jesus' disciples], the body of Christ is the Church, so when you share this common meal together, it is a recognition of Christians' interrelationship and unity with one another. Drawn together as a family, they become brothers and sisters together in Christ. This is often a closer bond than a blood relationship, because you have in common the spiritual beliefs that are essential in life: God's spirit in your life, and a love toward one another that is often deeper than the love that exists between family members."

John Dominic Crosson, Professor Emeritus of Religious Studies at DePaul University, refers to the taking of the Christian community meal among equals as an "open table."[13] As the early Christians expressed thanks over the bread and wine, broke the bread, and distributed both elements to those at the open table in their homes, they created a symbol for a new society. "In this manner the Sacrament was instituted, and from then on the act of breaking bread in the Gospels was closely related to the presence of Christ," writes theologian George Galavaris.[14]

Meal of Mystery

Of the mysterious qualities attributed to the bread and wine of the Eucharistic sacrament, writer Hans Beidermann tells us that Hildegard of Bingen wrote in the twelfth century: "'We cannot see that secret vital force...which gives life to the grape and the grain,'" yet, says Beidermann, "the same force is at work when the bread and wine of the Eucharist are transformed into the flesh and blood of Christ."[15]

What is it about the sacrament of bread and wine that holds such reverence—that has captured the imagination of Christians over the centuries? Of all the food served at the Last Supper, why did Jesus select bread and wine specifically to feed his followers after he would be gone? A closer look at the symbolic history of these elements may give us a clue.

Bread. When Jesus took bread and distributed it among his disciples during the Last Supper, the gesture held a multidimensional meaning. According to Hebrew tradition at the time, eating bread brought divine life and participation in the divine nature.[16] Indeed, as a source of sustenance for thousands of years, bread signified an essential, basic food, the "staff of life" that provided spiritual nourishment and sustenance for the human soul.

Yet after the Last Supper, controversy raged as to whether the bread Jesus used was leavened or unleavened. Based on a liturgical disagreement about the date of the Last Supper, regarding whether it occurred the day proceeding or on Passover, Eastern churches used leavened bread, while the Western Eucharistic rite included unleavened bread.[17]

The debate is significant, for unleavened bread is distributed during the Jewish Passover meal in remembrance of the quick exodus from Egypt when the Jews did not have time to let bread rise. If the Last Supper did *not* occur on Passover, then it is likely that Jesus and his followers consumed leavened bread. In addition, for early Jews, natural unleavened bread was seen as a gift from God, and therefore was believed to be holy; adding yeast would profane it, while fermentation symbolized corruption.[18] Indeed, in the New Testament, leavened bread continues to symbolize corrupting influences; this is evident when Paul tells the Corinthians to purge themselves of the yeast of evil, and to become the sincerity and truth attributed to leavened bread.[19]

In the Middle East during Jesus' time, the expression "to break bread together" evolved because portions of bread were broken off from the loaf rather than sliced. Historically, breaking bread had also been a custom used during ancient funeral rites as an offering to the lord of death.[20] Over time, it became a sacred observance that symbolized spiritual sustenance.[21] This is evident, when, after the Last Supper, "the entire process that culminates in bread—reaping, threshing, baking the processed grain from which the sacred bread is prepared—came to symbolize the Christian's laborious life on earth, which was to culminate in the blessed sanctity of heaven," writes Biedermann.[22]

Interestingly, because it was important for early Christians to hide their identity from the secular Romans, a system of secret bread codes evolved. Many Christians purchased bread at local bakeries that were baked in the shape of the cross, while other loaves were imprinted with specially designed stamps that identified it as Christian bread.[23]

Wine. In Jesus' time, wine was thick and strong; when he reached for the chalice, the red Passover wine it contained had been diluted according to custom: two parts of water to one of wine.[24] When wine is mixed with water, as it was during the Last Supper and during Holy Communion in early Christianity, the mixture symbolized the dual nature of Christ—both God and human being.[25] For Hebrews during the Passover feast, wine also represented the cup of blessings that symbolized God's promise of redemption: to deliver and redeem the Jewish people as a nation.[26]

Passing the wine-filled cup among his disciples, Jesus said,

"This cup that is poured out for you is the new covenant in my blood (Luke 22:20)." Says Dr. Harrop: "The wine is a symbol of Jesus' shed blood, perhaps in part because it is red. And of course, for Jews, because the blood was considered to be life itself, Jews were, and are, forbidden to consume blood." Indeed, because blood was life, to shed blood was to give life. And so the wine became a recognition for Jesus' having given his life for his people.

Wine as a sacrament is also believed to provide spiritual wisdom that is offered to God, says writer J. C. Kooper. "As the wine becomes the blood of the divinity," he writes, it is believed to impart "spiritual or vital power to the initiate."[27]

Merging Mystery with Science

The debate among Christians as to the nature of the power of the taking of the Eucharistic bread and wine is ongoing. Is transubstantiation symbolic or a profoundly true, divine mystery? Are Jesus' body and blood actually transmuted through consecrated bread and wine to be ingested by worshippers, or do they serve as a memorial to Jesus' divinity? Says Father Bryant: "By partaking in the Eucharist, we are bringing the past into the present, not just merely by remembering, but by re-entering Jesus' Godliness. Traditionally, the Latin expression for this is *hoc est enim corpus meum*: "This is my body." Adds Father Bryant parenthetically: "The expression *hocus pocus* evolved from this Latin expression, from those who said the medieval Mass was sacrilegious, magical," rather than a divine mystery wherein Jesus actually is made present in the sacrament of the church and worshippers are transformed into the grace of Christ in all aspects of their lives.

To grapple with the emergence of such lofty transubstantiation issues during the Middle Ages, the Catholic church, in part, turned to Aristotelian science, which was popular at the time. Based on Aristotelian "rational" beliefs, the church said that an authentic sacrament must include *matter* (such as the bread and wine); *form* (such as the recitation of specific prayers); and *right intention,* communicated by an ordained priest. With these three conditions met, the devotee could expect to receive the grace of the sacrament.[28]

During the twentieth century, theologians continued to grapple with the "magic (symbolic) vs. mystery (real)" debate. But with more sophisticated scientific knowledge and insights about how the universe is ordered, particularly with the more recent unfolding of quantum science, some theological writers, such as David S. Toolan, speculate that transubstantiation is a mystery that is actualized every time someone partakes of the Eucharist. For quantum theory leaves room for the possibility that consciousness may indeed affect matter such as bread and wine; therefore, the belief and intention to imbue the bread and wine with spirit actually changes it in some way.

Writes Toolan: "Matter (such as bread and wine) does as human beings do. It is not passive but active...repeatedly taking...material ... and converting it into something else. It is thus rich in promise. At one level or another, what Catholics call transubstantiation has been going on since the very beginning."[29] Toolan concludes that the universe is not comprised of separate entities; rather, he believes there is a "kinship" and unity of all matter, and thus everything is being affected by everything else all the time.

Such lofty concepts open the door to the possibility that the Eucharistic experience is more than symbolic; rather, that it is a true communing with the body of Christ, an experience of the manifestation of the abundance of God's love. One explanation may be that by ingesting the body and blood of Christ, Catholics infuse their cells with the physical manifestation of the love of God. By participating in the Eucharist, the love of God is not entering through the mind but directly into the cells of the body. For most Protestants, the word of God itself is God's direct communication with human beings; for Catholics, it occurs both through the word of God and by direct participation in the Eucharist.

Savoring the Eucharistic Community

Jean Molesky-Poz, a practicing Catholic and former member of a Franciscan religious community, had just such a "connection" when she was a child. Currently a lecturer in Ethnic Studies at the University of California, Berkeley, she told me about her first encounter with the Eucharist at age seven: "I was at a church in San Bruno, California, and had not yet taken my first Communion. But during a Eucharistic service, I actually remember feeling this overwhelming presence of being loved; that nothing would ever harm me, and that I would be held in that kind of love forever. I recall almost being taken into another time and place at that moment, of being filled with love. Something in my soul had been touched."

Carrying this memory and loving awareness into adulthood, Molesky-Poz joined the Franciscan religious community "to contribute to the world community and help to make a more just world." Her motivation? "As we share in the breaking of the bread...in that mystery... we're also sharing in the breaking of our own lives too. But the Eucharist is not only that event," she continues, "it is also the encounter that we have with other people. As we share words, I am also breaking my life, I am breaking open my memory and sharing it with others, and they with me."[30]

Reflecting on the strong communal aspect of the Eucharistic experience, Manetta Manetta says that "taking the Eucharist is an ordinary experience that is an expression of our community ordinariness. It recognizes that regardless of our differing customs, we all share our humanity and our dignity as people. It reminds us that we have a connectedness in spirit, that the Christ is the unifying symbol for how the word of God is to be interpreted and transformed into action" in both our everyday lives, as well as in the community.

Living a Eucharist "Consciousness"

After Christians have been with Jesus in the church, they "carry him immediately out into the world," writes Kevin Orlin Johnson, "because that's where he's needed."[31] Indeed, "Christianity and the Eucharist is not only about focusing inwardly," says Father Bryant, "it also has a lot to do with helping your neighbor...and putting ourselves in *relationship* at the core of our being" to others and God.

Says Molesky-Poz: "The commitment to Eucharist is a love for Jesus, but it's more than that. It's also a commitment to community. The Eucharist is an emotional and spiritual place to unite with others, to remember them, and in some way, to build a bond with one another. As a mother, this translates into love of my children, my husband, the students I teach, my colleagues...my awareness of people."

She continues: "I realize how important it is for me to be fed spiritually when I go to liturgy; I'm really hungry for this connection. With this in mind, I realize that students are also hungry in many ways, not just for information, but for knowledge and understanding relationships. The Eucharist consciousness actually changes me in terms of my ethical responsibility as an instructor—to provide, to nurture, to give enough food in terms of intellectual involvement. It's also behind my relating with students in both a just and compassionate way, with mercy."

Home Fellowship. Some Christians create a sense of community through weekly, personal, religious ceremonies. My in-laws, Jerry and JoAnna Scherwitz, are Christians who make their living through farming and ranching in a rural community in West Texas. For more than two years, in the tradition of the gathering of early Christians in private homes, they have been celebrating the Eucharist with other Christians through home fellowships. Here is Jerry's description of their Sunday spiritual gatherings.

"When we meet in our homes to partake of Holy Communion, we share an intimate remembrance of Christ and the sacrifices He made. By sharing in Communion, we're living in Christ's spirit; walking in the light that He shed before us.

"The home fellowship movement started in our community about four years ago. There are about twenty-five other home fellowships in our area that come together on Sunday mornings for worship service in our local civic center. The two-hour service is led by lay people, mostly Christians who are musically inclined. We meet for two hours on Sunday morning to worship, then smaller groups get together in various homes in the evening. We meet in our homes, just as the early Christians did until 313 AD. Our particular home fellowship consists of maybe fifteen or twenty people, ranging from five-years-old to teenagers and adults. We alternate homes, and each meeting begins at 5:00 pm and lasts until 9:00 or 10:00 PM.

"When we begin, we sit in a circle; some people sit on the floor; others sit on easy chairs and sofas. We always begin by introducing and recognizing guests. Then, after an icebreaker [some light conversation], we invoke the presence of the Holy Spirit by prayer. Here is an example:

> *Lord, we have gathered together here in your name*
> *To praise you in spirit and truth*
> *God, we want you to be with us*
> *To feel your presence, feel your power*
> *We want to experience your love anew and afresh.*
> *We want to experience your forgiveness.*
> *And Lord, we want to glean from your wisdom and your strength.*

"After the invocation, we praise and worship God through songs. In essence, we're dropping the secular and focusing on Christ through worship. We may do this for thirty or forty minutes, then someone may share scripture — something special that they had read during the week; someone else may share a teaching; another might share a testimony.

"Then we say prayers over the Lord's Supper. First we break a loaf of bread in half. Then we pass it around and each person tears off a small piece. We also pass around small cups, which hold grape juice. This can be done in silence or in song — depending on how the spirit leads us. When the last person has taken of the grape juice, we share a testimonial commentary about the forgiveness of sin and being made clean once again. We thank the Lord for this—that we've been made whole by His brokenness. Then we may sing again, worship, and say prayers that are from our hearts. This part of the service varies from week to week.

"After sharing Holy Communion, we break up into small groups of three or four, with each group going into different rooms in the house. At this point, the ministry becomes very intimate: some may confess a sin, share a hurt or concerns about school work; others discuss financial concerns, or illness. We lay hands on the person for whom we're praying. This part may last for thirty to sixty minutes.

"After, we share a potluck evening meal together—perhaps some fresh-caught catfish, or some homemade enchiladas or tamales prepared by a Mexican couple. The intention is to share the food within the body of Christ and to have intimate contact with our brothers and sisters. This way, we share food together every Sunday night the way the early Christians did.

"We believe that the bread is the body of Christ, and that the bread has Christ's power of healing—both the physical and spiritual infirmities; the wine holds the power of forgiveness of sins. Taking communion releases us spiritually from the bondage of sins. It brings us a sense of joy, peace, fulfillment, and thanksgiving, each day. Sins are not only forgiven, but blotted out. And the presence of the Holy Spirit makes us realize that Christ is in our heart."[32]

Sacred Sustenance

"When we take the Eucharist," says Father Bryant, "we place on the altar our broken words, our burdens, pains, suffering, passion, death—both little deaths and physical death—in the hope and knowledge of Christ having conquered death and made the whole creation new. That is what the Eucharist is: It's offering up to God and getting life back again—through food."

Participating in the Eucharist may take on even more significance when we reflect that Christianity is unique in that it is, in essence,

41

devoid of other food rules, the dietary guidelines that seem to permeate other major wisdom traditions. Dr. Harrop believes that "Christianity's absence of food-related rules comes from the seventh chapter of Mark's gospel, for it is here that Jesus is asked, 'From where does defilement come? From outside or from within?' And Jesus replies: 'Nothing that goes into a man from outside can pollute him' (Mark 7:15). Thus, He made all foods clean (Mark 7:19). We're told that what we eat isn't of primary importance; rather, what's inside is important: our commitment to God and the recognition that all good things come from God."

Such spiritual ideas inspire additional reflection about the taking of the Eucharist. What is it in our being that is capable of tasting and seeing and touching this sacrament? asks Caroline Walker Bynum, a professor of history at Columbia University. "The soul's sensitivity," she responds. "This eye sees in that whiteness (of the bread) the Divine nature joined with the human; wholly God, wholly human; the body, soul, and blood of Christ, his soul united with his body and his body and soul united with my divine nature."[33]

It is in the silent space between the soul and the ingestion of the bread and wine that the spiritual sustenance inherent in the Eucharistic ritual occurs. For in just such a transformative moment, does the mystery of the Holy Communion reveal itself. And as it does, so too may we catch a glimpse of God's great bounty of spiritual nourishment.

Communion Concepts

Following are suggestions from Father Robert Bryant, Jean Molesky-Poz, and Dr. Clayton Harrop for bringing the Eucharist's spiritual light into everyday food-related activities, no matter your spiritual orientation. Thomas Moore, author of *The Care of the Soul*, would explain such potentially transformative suggestions, insights, and reflections, as "lacing food with sacred imagination."[34]

Father Robert Bryant:

Create communion. "Focus on fellowship. A key aspect of the Eucharist is that it be done within a community of the faithful. Dine with others, and share your meals with family or friends."

Mind the nourishment. "Bring mindfulness to whatever it is that you're doing each moment. If you're doing physical work, stop and consider the food. Think about it. Look at the food. Where did it come from? What was involved in bringing this food to your table? Appreciate the food. While cooking or eating, avoid reading, watching television, listening to the radio, working on the computer, etc."

Give thanks. "Express thanks for the food, perhaps with prayer, which Father Bryant defines as "keeping us in relationship with God." The prayer he suggests is:

> *Holy God, as you feed me*
> *Spiritually with the Eucharist*
> *Remind me of the great sacrifice*
> *And the love of Jesus.*
> *Remind me of the sacrifice*
> *That which I now need."*

Slow down. "If you're in a hurry or meeting a deadline while you're eating, pause briefly. If you know you're going to eat quickly because of time constraints, thank God beforehand for the meal or snack: *Thank you, God. Next time I'll take more time.* Acknowledge that there will be another meal where you will be able to take the time to focus on the food."

Create a ritual. "*Rituals* are anything that connects us with the sacred and draws us closer to God, the higher power in our life; *worship* is about making *connections*, being in a holy state. Whether your meal is a sandwich or a more elaborate dining experience, one way to appreciate and connect to the food is through a ritual that engages all of your senses: sight, hearing, touch, smell, and taste."

Appreciate water. "A priest *blesses* (sets apart for the glory of God) Holy Water in the name of the church. Prayer, however, is designed to keep us in relationship with God, bring a sense of connectedness. Whenever you turn on the faucet to use water for cooking or coffee, express a brief prayer of appreciation."

Jean Molesky-Poz:

Dining. "Our family always eats together. I try to make the meal a nurturing experience by covering the table with a tablecloth, presenting food in an artistic, appealing way. And we try to encourage the sharing of stories while eating."

Cooking. "Eucharist influences some of my food preparation, because the act of Eucharist begins with breaking open our lives. To take time to care and prepare a nurtured and beautiful meal—this is also a breaking open of my being, my wisdom, my understanding, my technology, to provide for my family. Even the aroma of different foods is welcoming and satisfying."

Family. "My husband and I have a daughter who is eight. Our daughter is preparing for Eucharist this year. Occasionally we will develop a ritual on Sunday night to talk about the importance of bread and the sharing of bread and wine; sometimes we do art activities about the Eucharist. I feel my life as a mother is an extension of the Eucharist."

Dr. Clayton Harrop:

Fellowship meal. "We have a fellowship meal in the church every Wednesday night, cooked by some of the ladies in the church. Other groups may meet in different homes perhaps once a month with a potluck type of meal. My wife and I are part of a group of about ten people that does this, and we've been doing it for several years now.

"Sharing food and fellowship ultimately also has a lot to do with your relationship to God. John writes in the Gospel: 'You cannot love God whom you have not seen if you do not love your Brother whom you have seen.' If we cannot love one another here, how can we love God whom we have not seen?"

Spirit of gratitude. "Everything that is good in life is a gift from God, including the food we eat. We may have gone out and worked all week so that we could buy it, but God is the one who gave us the job, the strength or ability to work. So we recognize this always, and the best way to do this is to generate a spirit of gratitude for the food and all else He has given us.

"A professor of mine said that we don't bless the food; rather, we give thanks to God for the food. And we use the food to bless our lives. In regular prayers, there is a thanksgiving for all of the good that God gives, which would include food. Saying a prayer before a meal would go back to the Jewish practice of praying before eating and giving thanks to God."

Food for life. "It's wrong to eat something that is going to harm your body, because we're taught that our body is the temple of the holy spirit, and you do not defile the temple. Therefore, Christians ought to eat food that is healthy and good for them; food that builds up their body instead of destroying it."

four

African Roots:
American Soul Food

"Soul food, black folk cooking ... is compassion food
... and the act of eating 'soul' is ... to impart to food
a savor deep enough for joy and solace."[1]
—Soul food restaurateur
Pamela Strobel

With roots on the African continent, American *soul food* evolved from the suffering and sorrow of slaves on southern plantations. Motivated by the best of what is in the human heart, the creators of African American soul food triumphed by creating a culinary art that stretched simple foods and in the process transformed body and soul and helped the spirit soar. Today, this unpretentious fare— spiced with spirit, stirred with soul, and served "from the heart"—is a reminder of a culinary heritage that embraces simple flavors, places a high premium on kinship, community, and friends, and relishes reminiscences and remembrances. It is unique in that it is an oral culinary tradition that flavors food with care, a preference for freshness, and a deeply ingrained regard for those who will eat it. Following is a look into the essence of this true comfort food, and a visit with some of those who have mastered the art of cooking from the soul.

Dinner On the Ground

Surrounded by Secret Service agents, Vice President Al Gore looked at the various yogurts and fresh vegetables on the table in front of him. Then the Tennessee native's eyes lit on the fare being enjoyed by agents at a nearby table: pork chops smothered in onions, fried chicken, succotash (corn and lima beans), black-eyed peas, corn bread, and peach cobbler pie. "Do y'all mind if I go over there and have some of that kind of food?" he asked.

"That kind of food" was none other than soul food prepared by Adolf Dulan, proprietor of Aunt Kizzie's Back Porch restaurant, and his staff of forty-five. Located in a cozy nook in a shopping center in Marina del Rey, California, the atmosphere at Aunt Kizzie's literally crackles with good cheer. The name Kizzie, which means "stay put," comes from a character in *Roots*, the television miniseries; while "the 'back porch' signifies a place where you can be comfortable and relaxed," explains Dulan. "If you're in a little town and people pass by while you're sitting on the front porch, you're kind of at your best. But on the back porch, well, you can sit and spit watermelon seeds out in the yard."

The menu I hold in my hand says Aunt Kizzie's Back Porch serves soul food in the tradition of "all-American down-home Southern food just like Mother used to cook." Indeed, the menu is unfailingly *soul*. A sampling: "Uncle Wade's baked beef short ribs, which are lean and meaty and falling off the bone in brown gravy"; vegetables include "Aunt Gin's candied yams," "old-fashioned fresh collard greens," and "black-eyed peas." There are "old-time country desserts" such as "Miss Flossy's floating sweet potato pie, so light it can float like a feather." Explained Dulan, "These are recipes my wife, Mary, and I picked from different sides of our families."

All fare is billed as "old time dinner on the ground." "Have you ever heard of 'dinner on the ground?'" Dulan asked rhetorically, when I spoke with him at his restaurant. Just above our table hangs a photograph of a humble log cabin. Built in 1889, it was his parents' home when they lived in Missouri, although Dulan grew up in a rural community in Oklahoma. The photograph is one of more than 600 pictures adorning Aunt Kizzie's walls. Dulan is a tall, lanky man with intelligent features. Eloquent and elegant, with salt-and-pepper hair, he occasionally stopped our conversation briefly to greet customers.

"The expression 'dinner on the ground,' he explained, "began in the church. If there was a program there, such as a singing event, people would stay all day long. Then all the sisters [members of the church] would bring food for their family—and extra food to be shared by the minister, people from other churches ... whomever.

"The food would be placed on long tables so there would be this long line, and you'd get some of this dish and that dish, prepared by different people. And you'd have this big plate full of food. But because there wasn't a table to serve the food, it would be like it was picnic food, so we would have 'dinner on the ground.'"

Clementine "Clem" Bradshaw, seventy-eight years young, remembers such feasts from stories told to her by her mother about her mother's childhood in Pine Bluff, Arkansas. Today, Clementine is a homemaker living in Godfrey, Illinois. Reminiscing about the role food played in church gatherings, she reflects some of Dulan's memories. "Before desegregation, particularly in the south, black people weren't out in the street much ... entertaining each other, going to movies." Because of this, "sharing food at church provided one of the few chances we had to get dressed up and be with other people. The food was served outside on long tables; everybody would bring a favorite dish, and it was the highlight of the week."

Spiritual Survival

Soul food. Created with care and shared by family and friends, is a culinary tradition carved out by slaves as a creative expression of who they were as human beings. But for many, it was even more than that: it was also a means of resourcefulness, creative expression, and survival of both body and spirit. Writes sociologist Josephine A. Beoku-Betts: "The preparation and serving of food by Black women in a

secular communion of fellowship 'symbolize[s] the spiritual component of collective survival.'"[2]

Today, such spiritual fellowship is alive and well. Says Bradshaw:
"My mother's cooking was almost like magic. She put everything she
had into the food she made. Along with the ingredients, there was also
heart and soul and love and care. It's not about competition," she
notes, "we want to show we care." Says Dulan: "Few pleasures were
available to slaves. About the best thing you could do was sit down
with some friends and have something to eat."

Making Do

Having enough food to eat was a cause for celebration. *Soul Food*
author Sheila Ferguson tells us that typical slave rations of "something
to eat" consisted of "a peck of corn, three pounds of bacon or salt pork
a week, along with molasses, clabber (clotted milk), and small
amounts of seasonal fruit and vegetables."[3]

Other meager rations of leftover "slavery food" included "the pig
feet, and chitlins [pigs' intestines made into food]," adds Dulan. "In
order to stretch this, we had to find other things to cook. So we
learned how to go out into the woods and find edible wild greens, wild
onions, wild roots, wild potatoes, wild whatever.... And we would
bring our bounty back to the slave cabin, and mix it with the corn
bread and meal we had." If it was available, a bit of bacon or meat
drippings would be used as seasoning.

Although such "make do" foods were the staples from which
many soul food dishes evolved, such basics eventually grew into a cornucopia of foods, some of which made their way by sea to America
from Africa during the oceanic voyage that is sometimes called the
Middle Passage.

For instance, goobers (peanuts) brought from Africa found their
way into soups, stock, and sauces in meals prepared for the "big
house" on the plantations. Although in Africa garden-fresh peanuts
were served as a vegetable, "the inventiveness of soul cooks" on plan-

tations opened the door for such dishes as Kay's Yam Peanut Thing, we are told by author Evan Jones in *American Food: The Gastronomic Story*.[4] This is "a deep-fried dish made with chopped peanuts, mashed yams, eggs, crumbs, and seasonings [that are] formed into small cakes and stippled with shredded coconut" before they're fried.

Sesame seeds were another African staple. Although European cooks living in America used sesame seeds sparingly in some dishes, *benne* (the African word for sesame seeds) was native to African cooking. Pounded and made into a paste, *benne* was added to hominy, used to thicken soups, and as a flavor- and protein-enhancer.

Soul cooks also continued the African tradition of adding spices to transform simple dishes such as stews and succotash into tasty treats. Because they were so scarce and meager, meat and animal products were used as flavorings rather than as main courses. Consider Bradshaw's improvised recipe for string beans: "I'll tell you how I make 'em good. I get hog neck bones that have been smoked. Then I add a whole, small onion, a garlic button, and salt and pepper. I cook the neck bones a little bit first...and then simmer the beans with the smoked neck bone, so the smoked flavor gets into the beans. I cook it on a low flame for about an hour, or until the beans are tender. Before I serve it, I take out the neck bones, onion, and garlic button. And sometimes I put white potatoes on top."

Beyond the Basics

To learn more about authentic soul food, Beoku-Betts visited the African American Gullah communities in the Sea Islands of Georgia and South Carolina.[5] Many of the residents are descendants of formerly enslaved Africans who began living on the islands in the 1600s. Because of the isolation of these islands, many African cultural traditions have been preserved—more so than that of other groups of African Americans living in the United States.

Today, Gullah food—as is typical of soul food from other parts of America—is a crosscultural mixture of European, Native American, and African American cuisines. As with other soul food throughout the south, both *how* it's prepared and the *type* of seasonings that are used are what makes it unique. Beoku-Betts offers these reflections by Velma Moore, a member of the Gullah community: "We are a make-do society...because, as with slaves in the past, you can't run to the supermarket to get things. We are plain cooking. We use salt, pepper, and onion as basic additives. Our flavoring comes from the type of meat we put in it...pig tails, neck bones, and ham hock is what we use. Soul food is what other Americans call it, but we consider these to be foods we always ate."[6]

Along with spices and flavorings, other soul food basics include a potpourri of fresh vegetables such as turnip and squash; fruits such as watermelon (the seeds of which were also brought to America from Africa); and grains such as rice and corn. It also includes squirrel, possum, fresh fish, and wild game. Says Dulan: "We took these simple foods and turned them into a delicacy, something that tasted good. I believe that by creating this food, we had something that was our own, that we had made. And because it wasn't written down, nobody could reproduce it."

Cooking from "Feel"

In lieu of writing down recipes (slaves were not allowed to learn to read or write), fresh ingredients, seasonings, and ongoing tasting became important components of a successful soul food dish. Creating soul-satisfying food also came to depend on improvisation, approaching the food with patience, and coaxing it along with lots of love. As with any art, soul food is not something that can be slapped together or rushed. Instead, it calls for what both Dulan and Bradshaw describe as "cooking from feel."

"About 95 percent of the time, I can go into our kitchen and just by looking at something, can tell you if it tastes right. I can tell just by the *feel* of it," says Dulan. He told me that to make good soul food, along with certain ingredients, you must use your senses. You taste it, listen to when it's boiling or crackling, or sense when it smells done. Bradshaw also uses her sixth sense to cook: "My mother taught me how to make cornbread without any recipes. But now I know how to make it by 'feel.'"

And, as with any art, when one person makes something, it may be lifeless; but someone else might create the same dish with depth and it will speak to your heart. Making soul food "is like jazz," said Dulan. "As you know, jazz is a contribution from Afro-Americans. Many years ago, there was no written score for this music. So you could play the same song, but it might never be played the same way twice." It's all in how it's improvised.

Intuiting what will work in a dish is a major aspect of making soul food with "heart." Mrs. Bradshaw says she watched her mother cook until she developed her own intuitive feel for what works—and what doesn't. Today, when she tastes a dish she likes—or doesn't—she'll go home and create her own version. When she raised her two children and served them meals, she said she extended the pleasing aspects of the meal by creating spirited ways to serve it. For instance, she would vary the colors of the food (green broccoli, orange carrots), so that the presentation would be visually pleasant.

Cooking, Community, and Kin

Along with serving as an expression of creativity, soul food also offered comfort to heart, body, and soul in another major way: it provided a joyous opportunity to connect with others and spend time with family and friends. Says author Evan Jones: "To be able to cook and feed children and friends was more often than not one of the few real pleasures that black families could share. It was also a way to exercise creative urges.... Mostly it was a way of feeling free."[7]

What is it about soul food that is so satisfying? Clara Oliver, a cook at Aunt Kizzie's Back Porch, says soul food is gratifying because it's "cooking that comes from the soul. It comes from what you know, what your grandmother taught you. It's good because it's cooked with love."

Echoing Oliver's sentiments, Bradshaw says, "My mother was an outstanding cook, even though she didn't have much money or food to cook with. I think her food was so good because of the love she put into it." Like mother, like daughter: Bradshaw is carrying on a tradition that is hundreds of years old. "I put my heart, soul, and love into the food I make," she says. "I care how it comes out."

To highlight soul food's unique blend of "feel" and intuition, and the inherent joy of sharing it with kin and community, Dulan told me a story about a recent family reunion. "Just before a 'get-acquainted' party for all the relatives, we needed some cooked dishes for everybody to eat. My seventy-five-year-old sister Celia remembered a casserole dish she used to cook that included chicken and dressing. And then I recalled a similar dish, made with vegetables and chicken cooked together—a great big casserole dish. Then Celia suggested we go to Aunt Kizzie's to see if we could create it.

"So we came here to the restaurant, and I gathered some fresh broccoli, cauliflower, carrots, celery, and onions. I mixed them together, then put them in the pan. Then my sister added a layer of chicken. Another layer of vegetables went on top of that; then another layer of chicken. Then Celia topped it with cornbread stuffing.

"And then we thought about some soup...cream of mushroom soup, and cream of chicken.... So we went to the store, got the soups ... and added them. Next, Celia remembered a dish made with olives that tasted good. So I went to the store again, bought green olives, sprinkled them over the top....

"By this time, the casserole was this long and this deep." Demonstrating his point, he simulates the shape of the casserole dish with his hands. "Then we cooked it in the oven for forty-five minutes— until the vegetables got to just beyond crunch.

"That baby came out of there bubbling hot, and it was the hit of the evening. People asked for the name of it. They wanted the recipe, too. Well, there's no name, and there's no recipe."

Does cooking from the heart—cooking with care—make a difference? According to Mr. Dulan, it does. "If you gave ten people a brush, paint, and canvas and the same picture to paint, you'll probably come up with ten different pictures. But one will be better than the others...because of something they drew on from within themselves."

That "something" is an ability to invest food with enough soul to transform "nothing into something." Another "something": sharing your bounty of simple food with others and, in the process, bringing a palate-pleasing smile to their whole being—body, heart...and soul.

Secrets of Soul Cooks

Dulan's odyssey into the heart of soul food cooking began when, as the youngest of two sisters and one brother, he was assigned cooking "detail" by his mother. Over time, he "began to pick up how to make rolls with yeast, biscuits, cornbread, homemade ice cream, and other dishes." As a matter of fact, a family joke developed around his cooking expertise. "You could wake me up in the middle of the night, and I could recite the recipe: one cup of flour, one cup of meal, one teaspoon of sugar, one teaspoon of salt, two eggs..." he recalls, a smile reaching his eyes. "Nothing was written down. My mother didn't give me a recipe. You just did it."

Just "doing it"—making your own soul-satisfying food—calls for tapping into what we've learned from the oral teachings of African American mothers and grandmothers over the centuries. What follows is a synthesis of key concepts you'll need to capture the essence of soul food cooking in your kitchen. Of course, they're "recipeless." This is because the most important ingredients are not the foods in the dish, but the heartfelt attitude and loving intention you mix into the meal you make.

Stay sincere. Soul food is *not* about frills and turning unpretentious fare into fancy food. Should you decide to include an ingredient or add a sauce, do so only because these "extras" will enhance the taste of the dish and satisfy the palate. Don't add ingredients because you "should" or because "that's how it's always done."

Improvise intuitively. Centuries ago in Africa, it was common to walk outside and gather food for a dish from a nearby field. The tradition carried over to plantation life, when slaves would scour the country- side seeking wild vegetables and game. Be spontaneous. A little bit of this and a little of that—based on what's available, and what you *sense* would work well in the dish—is what soul cooking is all about.

Season smartly. The dictionary tells us that *smart* can mean "amus- ingly clever; witty."[8] Indeed, stretching meager meals and poor qual- ity food calls for nothing less than bringing a sense of inventiveness and cleverness to how such food is flavored. Explore the tastes that various spices and herbs can create, and flavors that assorted sea- sonings can release.

Create comfort. Above all, approach the food you're cooking with care and love. "Good [soul food] cooks worked with their whole heart, doing the best they could with what they had on hand to make sure that their dishes would be enjoyed by all who sat down to eat,"[9] writes Evan Jones. Ask any good soul food cook: including a pinch of love is the secret to "doin' it right."

five

India: Yogic Nutrition

Beloved Mother Nature
You are here on our table as our food.
You are endlessly bountiful,
benefactress of all.
Please grant us health and strength,
wisdom and dispassion
to find permanent peace and joy.[1]

—ancient Sanskrit prayer

How steeped in dietary wisdom India is! Perhaps more than any other country, India's great traditions and religions are filled with food celebrations and ceremonies, myths and magic. What follows is a journey into the yogic world of **Sanatana dharma,**[2] the Sanskrit expression for the underlying, eternal, true essence of all religions. By following such a philosophy, yogis do not separate food from Self, God, or Nature, and turn all eating into a potentially sacred activity, each encounter with food into an opportunity to meet the Higher Self.

The Yoga of Food

Sitting at her circular dining table, Nischala Devi is almost ready to begin eating lunch. Breathing rhythmically, her breath peacefully ebbing and flowing, she carefully considers the simple vegetarian meal in front of her. A moment of meditation follows, allowing her to enter a consciousness of thankfulness and respect for the food. In a calm, focused frame of mind, she acknowledges that the food in front of her is a gift from Mother Nature. Next she closes her eyes, savoring the scent of the herbs that flavor the vegetable stew. Then, surrounded by silence and serenity, in awe of the food's life-giving abilities, she takes the first spoonful of her meal.

For more than twenty-five years, Devi has practiced *anna* yoga, the yoga of food. Summoned by a desire to lead a simpler life and "find herself," her commitment to yoga (which means "union") and its nutrition philosophy blossomed further after she joined the Integral Yoga Institute, an *ashram* (spiritual community), where people come together to enhance their own spirituality and serve humankind.

Devi's odyssey into yoga began in her early twenties when she was known as Joy Kraft and still lived in Philadelphia, her hometown. As her interest in the yoga lifestyle grew, so did her commitment to it. Eventually she became a swami (Monk) and adopted the name Nischalananda. In Sanskrit, *Nischala* means steadiness, calmness, serenity; *ananda* describes one who knows the self, bliss, or peace. Today she is married, uses the name Nischala Devi (*Devi* is the feminine aspect of light, or being of light), and no longer lives within the structure of an ashram.

I spoke with Devi about yogic nutrition at her hillside home in Northern California. As we talked, her glistening, prematurely silver hair reflected the wisdom in her words: "The yogic diet is a part of yoga's deep, deep spiritual well. Like the other systems of yoga, it is designed not only to nourish the body, but by encouraging us to bring a loving consciousness to our food, it also nourishes the mind and spirit, which, according to yogic philosophy, are not separate."[3]

Loving Nourishment

Perhaps more than any other food philosophy, the yogic diet is a repository of love-filled wisdom, designed to calm the mind and prepare the body to receive nourishment. According to O. M. Aivanhov in *Living Yoga: A Comprehensive Guide for Daily Life*, "eating is a magic rite during which the food becomes transformed into health, force, love, light. While you eat...think of...food with love, for that will make it open its treasures to you."[4]

The *Bhagavad Gita* ("The Song of the Blessed Lord"), is an epic poem about the various aspects of yoga and it includes a philosophy of nutrition. Believed to have been written about 300 BC, the *Gita* tells us that imparting a consciousness of love to food is an integral aspect of the spiritual path. In Sanskrit, *prana* is the word that describes this loving energy. *Prana* keeps us alive; it is the force of life that is in the food we eat, the air we breathe, everything.

Given that food's *prana*—its subtle, vital, life-giving quality—is a major consideration in yogic nutrition, the person cooking the food plays an important role. "The *Bhagavad Gita* tells us that if the cook who prepares the food is not of a loving, calm nature, the food won't benefit you—spiritually, mentally, or physically," says cardiologist Dr. K. L. Chopra.[5] An eloquent speaker who exudes intelligence and refinement, Dr. Chopra, chief of the Department of Medicine and Cardiology at the Mool Chand K. R. Hospital in New Delhi, India, has followed a yogic diet his entire life. I spoke with him during a break at the First International Conference on Lifestyle and Health in New Delhi.

Swami Dharmananda, a spiritual teacher at the Adhyathma Sadhana Kendra Yoga Center in New Delhi, describes the *Bhagavad Gita* as "one of yoga's main scriptures—a holy book that contains a nutritional approach for pursuing a spiritual life."[6] I spoke with him around dusk on the evening before the conference was to begin. He is a tall man with a melodious voice and gentle eyes that shine with playfulness when he speaks.

To pursue the spiritual life, he explains, "the *Bhagavad Gita* tells us to honor all living things—including food—as part of an interdependent oneness. With this consciousness, we are doing something that brings peace, bliss, and a stress-free life. This is how I perceive spirituality. And in India, as you become more deeply involved in spiritual growth, then you become a yogi, and you are supposed to take only yogic food."

Yogic Nutrition

What are "yogic foods"? One verse in the *Bhagavad Gita* tells us they are "foods that promote life, mental strength, vitality, cheerfulness, and a loving nature" (Chapter 17, verse 8). The *Bhagavad Gita* is a repository of wise words, but what makes its nutrition philosophy a coherent whole is the concept of the three *gunas*, or qualities of nature, mentioned throughout. Explains Swami Dharmananda: "It is written in our scriptures that the *gunas* are the three attributes of nature that reflect temperament, or inner life." Described in *Living Yoga*, here are the *Bhagavad Gita*'s perceptions of the three types of food—and qualities—associated with the *gunas* (Chapter 17, verses 8–10):

Sattvic
Foods that promote life, lucidity, strength, health, happiness, and satisfaction, and that are savory, rich in oil, firm, and heart-gladdening are agreeable to the sattva-natured person.

Rajasic
Foods that are pungent, sour, salty, spicy, sharp, harsh, and burning are coveted by the rajas-natured person.

Tamasic
That which is spoiled, tasteless, putrid, stale, left over, and unclean is food agreeable to the tamas-natured person.[7]

It is *sattva*, or *sattvic* food, that constitutes the yogic diet. To the Western mind, it is lacto-vegetarian, consisting mainly of fruits, vegetables, whole grains, beans and peas, nuts and seeds, and dairy products, particularly milk and yogurt. Honey, pure water, and *ghee* (clarified butter) are also believed to promote the *sattva* aspect. Eggs, which are perceived as *rajasic*, are avoided; because milk and yogurt are considered easy to digest, they are included. Where does cheese fit into this belief system? "If the cheese is soft and fresh, such as many of the cheeses in France, then it is considered *sattvic* and acceptable," offers Devi. "But aged cheeses can move into the *tamasic* category. Along with being old and moldy, aged cheeses are made from enzymes from the stomach of a cow, which would not be considered part of the yogic diet."

As a contrast, *rajas*, or *rajasic*, stimulating foods, such as coffee, chili peppers, garlic, and onions, are said to agitate and stimulate the mind and body. *Tamas*, the *tamasic* category, includes old or stale food, foods that are past their time that might have been in the pantry or refrigerator for a while, such as old crackers or frozen meat or poultry. According to the *Bhagavad Gita*, these foods are believed to promote laziness, allergies, and fatigue.

Because yogis believe that what we eat affects the mind, they suggest avoiding the extremes of tamasic and rajasic foods. "I like to think of the gunas as a seesaw," says Devi. "On one side you have *tamas*, the state of inertia, a lack of energy; the other side is *rajas*, an aggressive, overactive state. In the center of the seesaw is *sattva*, which is the balance between the two. This is the yogic diet. It is even, gentle, calming, promoting tranquility. When people practice yoga, they pursue a certain level of stillness in the body and mind. That's why they choose the *sattvic* diet."

Mending the Mind-Body

Along with creating food with loving energy, and recognizing that different foods promote different emotional states, the *sattvic* diet also places much importance on other of its mind-body benefits. "Because *sattvic* nutrition is natural and easily digested," explains Swami

Dharmananda, "you get only the nutrients that help the body...and the soul. When we take *sattvic* food, we feel less anger, greed, or jealousy—all these [negative] things the mind creates." What happens when we eat *rajasic* or *tamasic* foods? "Our contention is that if you eat spicy *rajasic* food, or *tamasic* food such as meat, fish, or poultry, digestion is more difficult. Then toxins have more of an opportunity to enter the bloodstream—not unlike the minerals from fruit that go inside the body, but now there are toxins. Organs can be affected by these impurities circulating in the blood. And if they are, we become ill."

With a focus on the digestive process, the *Bhagavad Gita* also suggests *when* to eat. "One should eat only when one is hungry, not when one thinks one should," advises Dr. K. L. Chopra. His rationale: eating when you're not hungry places a strain on the digestive system; in turn, this creates two problems. First, if you overeat you can stretch the stomach, and digestive enzymes then won't have room to digest the food with the result that the brain and heart get less nourishment. Second, overeating impairs circulation, increasing the odds of becoming sleepy afterward.

The *mentality* we bring to food is yet another important component for creating spiritual and physical well-being. "I try never to sit down to a meal without being thankful," says Devi. "I feel that if I don't give respect to the food I'm eating, it won't heal and nurture me." Respect is given, in part, by concentrating on the food: seeing it, then eating, chewing, and grinding it, making sure it's ready to be swallowed and put into the stomach.

One unique way to honor and respect food is by savoring its colors. In Europe where Devi taught yoga for many years, "many people first eat with their eyes," she recalls. "The food and natural colors are often arranged beautifully, so the eyes appreciate it first. Then the nose smells the food and digestion has already begun."

Roots of Spiritual Nutrition

Today, as director of stress management at the Preventive Medicine Research Institute (PMRI) in Sausalito, California, Devi teaches and trains yoga teachers at hospitals that are implementing PMRI's heart-healthy "reversal" lifestyle, based on the work of Dean Ornish, M.D., and colleagues. What Devi is teaching carries on a tradition that began nearly 4,000 years ago in the dense woods of India. It was there that *rishis* (seers), the original yoga practitioners, recorded their mystical insights, intuition, and wisdom in the *Upanishads*.

Since their creation thousands of years ago, the *Upanishads* have journeyed into today's world through texts and scriptures, eventually becoming a basis for later Hindu philosophy espoused in the *Bhagavad Gita*, Patanjali's *Yoga Sutras* (a second-century text that codified yoga philosophy), and other ancient texts. But it is the *Bhagavad Gita* that created a clear, concise nutrition philosophy capable of either impeding or speeding spiritual progress.

To perceive the *sattvic* diet described in the *Bhagavad Gita* only as a group of dietary rules and regulations, though, is to lose its essence and purpose. Evolved from the insights and intuition of spiritual seekers to enhance spiritual well-being, it promises to reveal levels of consciousness unfamiliar to most people. Indeed, with its mystical, anecdotal, experiential beginnings, the *Gita* presents itself as a guiding light for the nourishment of body, mind, and soul.

Linking nutrient-dense, nourishing foods such as fresh fruits and vegetables, whole grains, legumes, nuts, and seeds to spiritual well-being is based on the centuries-old practice of yogis using their own bodies and minds as laboratories. Over time, as their intuition, perceptions, and sensitivity became finely honed, they were able to detect in their own bodies energetic states of which others were unconscious.

Says Devi: "Yogis found that certain foods would tend to deposit toxins in the body, making it difficult to be still, to sit quietly and meditate, or to maintain certain poses. These ancient seers saw the *sattvic*, *rajasic*, or *tamasic* nature of food as based on its *vibrational* quality. This refers to the energy of the food. How powerful is that energy? Is it still life-giving?"

She offers the example of fruit ripened on a tree. "If you pick an apple from a tree, it has a certain quality *(prana)*, a certain energy within. If you take the same apple and cook or bake it, then its vibrational quality changes; it no longer has the same vitality. For a yogi, the vitality and energy in food is important, especially when you consider the diet's main purpose, which is to keep the body free from toxins and the mind quiet."

Within the framework of *sattvic* nutrition, the vibrational qualities of food take on supreme importance. *Sattvic* food is believed to nurture and heal, to sustain life. In contrast, *tamasic* or *rajasic* food may offer inadequate energy, therefore taking—rather than giving—life-sustaining energy.

Manifesting Spiritual Treasures

While *information* about vitamins and minerals, etc., is the core of Western nutrition, *transformation* is the essence of India's yogic-based nutrition philosophy. Like all yoga practices, the *sattvic* diet is designed to keep the mind tranquil. For only in a state of serenity, the yogis tell us, can our unique spirit emerge. Indeed, by encouraging us to linger in that limitless space between thought and breath, the yogic diet holds the promise of spiritual, physical, and emotional well-being.

Today, yoga's *sattvic* food philosophy, whose intuitive seeds were planted thousands of years ago by *rishis* meditating in India's ancient forests, continues to impart its wisdom. Through its surviving scriptures, it tells us that the relationship between ourselves and food is a gracious one. It asks us not to take more than we need; to acknowledge that what is being placed in front of us to eat is a gift from Nature. And through that food, we are able to function on this planet, thriving and growing, creating a conscious body-mind.

"If we know how to listen, food speaks to us," writes O.M. Aivanhov. "Food is condensed light and sound, but if your thoughts are busy elsewhere, you cannot hear the voice of the light."[8] India's ancient scriptures show us how to access the life-giving properties of food. It is up to us to listen to the message in our meals and, in the process, discover their spiritual treasures.

In Search of Spiritfood

What follows is a synthesis of dietary guidelines gleaned from India's ancient scriptures: the *Upanishads, Bhagavad Gita,* Patanjali's *Yoga Sutras,* and others. Developed by Swami Sivananda of Rishikesh, an ashram-filled town in the foothills of the Indian Himalayas, they are designed to help transform meals into an opportunity for spiritual growth. Himself a proponent of *Vedanta* yoga (a form derived from the *Vedas,* a body of ancient songs and texts), Swami Sivananda encouraged his disciples to practice all yogas and then assimilate their wisdom. In the same spirit, one should strive to approach the guidelines as dietary options, not dogma.

Vivian Worthington, author of *A History of Yoga,* tells us that before Sivananda died, he was quoted as saying, "I have sown my seed all over the world. It will sprout at the right time."[9] Synthesized by the Integral Yoga Institute,[10] here are some of Swami Sivananda's suggestions for "sprouting" *sattvic* wisdom in your own spiritual kitchen.

Consciousness While Eating

Always have love and respect for your food. The consciousness, or mentality, we bring to food may be the most important ingredient in the meal. Think positive thoughts of peace and love when preparing food. Such a consciousness may be transferred into the food, enhancing digestion, and empowering it with the ability to nourish both mind-body and soul.

Do not eat when angry. Negative thoughts are believed to create poisons that eventually are secreted by the glands. Like vitamins and minerals in life-giving foods, negative, angry thoughts may be metabolized, too, eventually producing toxins. Also, anger or stress may limit the production of digestive enzymes in our stomach, making it difficult for food to be adequately digested.

Take meals in a relaxed frame of mind. A calm state of mind is ideal for preparing the body to receive nourishment. During meals, silence or warm conversation among family members or friends can create balanced, loving energy, enhancing digestion and, ultimately, food's ability to nourish. Avoid eating when rushed.

Remember the Absolute, the life-force, the in-dweller of all foods. *Brahman* is the Sanskrit word that attempts to describe the indescribable; "a supreme, blissful consciousness" only hints at its meaning. Such a noble frame of mind is believed to make all but poisonous food healing, *sattvic,* and healthful. A verse from the *Bhagavad Gita* (4:24) expresses it this way:

> *The process of eating is Brahman;*
> *the offering [of food] is Brahman.*
> *The person offering is Brahman,*
> *and the fire is also Brahman.*
> *Thus by seeing Brahman everywhere in action,*
> *he [alone] reaches Brahman.*

Do not be a slave to any diet theory. Maintaining a mind that is tranquil and peaceful, pursuing union with the Absolute, is the purpose of all yoga. Following rigid dietary rules is more likely to produce the antithesis: stress, anxiety, worry, and doubt. Like the yogis, use your own experience and intuition to create your own ideal eating style.

What to Eat

Choose foods that promote a balanced state. To pursue physical and psychospiritual well-being, choose fresh, whole foods in their natural state as often as possible. Eat a natural diet that includes lots of fresh fruits, vegetables, whole grains, legumes, nuts, and seeds.

Avoid fried food. Centuries before knowledge of health-robbing free-radicals and fear of fat, yogis believed that fried food caused injury to the body. They were right. We now know that too much fat can impair the immune system, and is linked with heart disease and other ailments. Another reason to avoid fried food: it's considered *rajasic* and therefore hinders spirituality.

Select perfectly ripe fruit; avoid unripe fruits. Fruit that hasn't matured hasn't reached its nutritional peak. Not only is it difficult for your body to digest and assimilate, you'll also be cheating yourself nutritionally.

Liquids. Do not drink water or other liquids during, just before, or after meals. Though it is an unpopular idea in the West, liquids mixed with food are believed to dilute gastric juices, causing indigestion. The ideal: Drink liquids an hour or two before or after eating solid food. (*Note*: If you experience thirst while eating, moisten food with saliva. Chew food until solids becomes liquified in your mouth.)

Avoid drinking coffee or tea, especially at night. Coffee and tea contain caffeine, making them stimulating and *rajasic*. To maintain a serene state of mind—and sleep deeply—avoid beverages laced with caffeine.

When to Eat

Beware of false hunger. Eat only when you are truly hungry. A sensation of hunger is the body's built-in clock, telling you it's time to eat. If you "wait out" the desire to eat, and it leaves, then you're probably not really hungry. More likely, you're responding to eating cues or a habitual eating pattern. When you're truly hungry, the desire to eat will not go away.

Consume larger meals earlier in the day; eat lightly in the evening. Not only do we need—and use more efficiently—food energy eaten earlier in the day, but heavy evening meals are likely to cause weight gain. Why? Your body's metabolism, including digestion, slows down as the day progresses, even more so as you sleep. Try to make lunch the calorie-dense meal.

Avoid eating between meals or late at night. When you are truly hungry, meaning you have a good appetite, it's likely your stomach is "empty." Eating between meals or before going to sleep increases the odds that food from a prior meal hasn't been completely digested.

The result: Food may ferment, become acidic, or cause gas and bloating. To avoid this, do not eat at least two hours after a meal or before going to sleep.

How to Eat

Chew food thoroughly. The digestion of food begins in your mouth, when it mixes with enzymes in your saliva. Chew each mouthful slowly and thoroughly, until it is almost liquified. Avoid gulping down food; instead, swallow it slowly.

Stop eating when three-quarters of the stomach is full. Ancient scriptures tell us that the stomach is about as large as what you can hold in your two hands; perhaps about the size of your fist. The belief: filling your stomach about three-quarters during a meal leaves enough room for digestive enzymes to break down food. Overeating *sattvic* foods can make them *tamasic*.

Avoid eating food you do not enjoy — or overeating food you especially like. The mentality you bring to food is believed to influence the mind-body. Eating food you like increases the odds of imbuing it with positive, loving energy; food you do not enjoy is more likely to produce negative, "life-taking" vibrations. But even with *sattvic* foods you enjoy, moderation and balance are the keys.

Abandon too many food mixtures or combinations. Yogis place much importance on the stomach's digestive capacity, and eating according to what it can easily metabolize. They believe it is difficult for the body's digestive juices to digest complex food combinations. Eat only four or five kinds of food at any one meal.

six

Islam: Devout Dining

In Islam, eating is considered to be a matter of
worship of God, like prayers.[1]
—*Ahmad H. Sakr, Ph.D.*

The Prophet taught that . . . the consumption of
wholesome food . . . [is a] religious obligation.[2]
— *"Understanding Islam
and the Muslims"*

What a reverential, pious appreciation Muslims have for food!
Inherent in the Islam religion is the concept of **Ihsan,** the highest level
of faith that encourages devout Muslims to behave in their daily life
as if God is in front of them at all times—including in the food they
eat. To enhance this essential value, Muslims honor the dietary laws
set forth in Islam's sacred scripture, the **Qur'an** (also spelled Koran or
Coran), by God through the Prophet Muhammad in the sixth century, as well as the prophetic traditions and etiquette guidelines written about in the **Hadith.**

Because Muslims are asked to approach food with a heartfelt
awareness of God's great bounty, each dining experience becomes a
sacred opportunity to eat for **Allah,** the Supreme Being in Islam.
Especially during **Ramadan,** when millions of Muslims throughout the
world abstain from food, the sense of gratefulness for the divine gift
that is food is heightened.

From Fast to Feast

It is the holy month of Ramadan, and American Muslims Ameena Jandali, her husband, teenage daughter, and son—along with millions of other devout Muslims throughout the world—are fasting, observing the scripture, and praying from dawn to sunset. I spoke with Jandali at her spacious home in El Cerrito, California. Her handsome features communicate intelligence; the scarf that covers her head reflects a basic Islamic belief that women should remain covered, with the exception of their face and hands.

During this sacred month, the ninth in the Muslim lunar year, Muslims glorify God through the self-purification brought about by fasting. By denying themselves food and drink between dawn and dusk each day for one month, they gain sympathy for the hungry as well as achieve personal spiritual growth.[3]

It is also believed that fasting during Ramadan quiets both the spirit and the passions, provides a sense of unity to all Muslims, and gives them an opportunity to make amends for the sins of the past year.[4] Those unable to fast for various reasons (pregnancy, illness, etc.), participate in the spirit of Ramadan by feeding the poor and hungry each day.

During this time throughout the world, Muslim women prepare special nighttime meals for themselves, their families, friends, and neighbors. Different Muslim cultures may create different meals. For instance, based on local tradition, some Iranian Muslim women may prepare a different "round" of dishes for each night of Ramadan. However, all Muslims always avoid cooking or eating meals prepared with pork because of Islam's dietary code. This is a special challenge for Chinese Muslims, as pork is a prevalent food throughout China.[5]

Throughout this holy month, most Muslims break the daytime fast *(Iftar)* of Ramadan with savory dates—a food that is recommended by Allah—and water or milk because it is an easily metabolized liquid. In Ameena Jandali's family, the fast is also broken with assorted fruit and a light soup. "I usually cut up some fresh fruit, some organic oranges, perhaps some apples," she says. "Then I arrange the dates and fruit on a platter and serve them along with soup [such as lentil] that is easily digested.

"Before we break the Ramadan fast each day after sunset, we say a prayer. In our family, as we sit around our dining table, we each say the prayer separately. It may be said quietly, loudly, or in silence—from one's heart:

Oh God, I have fasted for you
And I have believed in you
And I have broken my fast
With your sustenance.

"After I say the prayer, I'll reach for some dates that are positioned closest to me on the platter, while at the same time my husband and children may select some nearby dates before helping themselves to other fruit. Usually other family members or friends are also present. Conversation is typical." Needless to say, "after fasting during daylight hours, the dates taste so very good."

After this initial "break of the fast," the family members perform five evening prayers together, expressing appreciation to Allah for all He has provided. "During our prayers at home, we are reminded that everything we have...is from God," explains Jandali, "and that everything will go back to God. This includes food, which is a blessing from God. After fasting for a month, food tastes so wonderful; we really appreciate God's dual blessing of food and drink."[6]

After the evening prayers are said, Jandali serves supper to her family and any guests who might have been invited over for the evening meal. Before eating, though, devout Muslims express appreciation for the food before them. Ahmad H. Sakr, Ph.D., founder of the Foundation for Islamic Knowledge, related to me the following prayers of appreciation, which are said throughout the year both before and after eating.

Before eating:

In the name of God,
The most merciful, the most gracious
Oh Allah, Bless the food that we eat
And the liquid that we drink
And make us happy, healthy,
And obedient servants to You.

After eating, the following prayer is recited:

Praise thee to God
For allowing us to eat, drink, and be satisfied
With the food and the liquid
We are grateful to Allah
That He made us obedient servants to Him.
That we have obeyed Him, come to Him, and submitted to Him.

Guests express appreciation to Allah for the food, and Jandali and her family for its preparation, with the following prayer:

Your food will be eaten by those who have been fasting
  (or are hungry)
We are among those good friends
Having been invited by you
We are thankful to you
The angels have made their prayers
For you to God, Almighty Allah
And Allah Himself is now acknowledging your favor upon us.[7]

Dishes Jandali has prepared include Middle Eastern fare: perhaps a Syrian dish called feta, which consists of pita bread covered with yogurt, garlic, sesame "butter" *(tahini)*, lemon, pieces of lamb, and pine nuts; salad; and other dishes, depending on whether guests are present, as they commonly are during Ramadan. After eating, the family will go to the local mosque for additional nighttime prayers and a special Ramadan prayer called *Taraweeh*.

Breaking the Fast

The last ten days of Ramadan are considered especially holy, for angels are believed to descend to Earth during this time with blessings for humankind. During the last night, the Night of Power *(Lailat al-Qaдr)*, traditionally celebrated on the twenty-seventh night of Ramadan, the angels are thought to be "bearers of Divine mercy," explains Hamid Algar, Ph.D., professor of Islamic Studies at the University of California, Berkeley. On this particular night, "[the angels] carry the prayers of devout Muslims [back] to God."[8] It is an evening that recalls the descent of the *Qur'an* from heaven, when its contents were first revealed to Muhammad by the Archangel Jibril *(Gabriel)* in the sixth century.[9] Adds writer John F. Wrynn, "It is traditionally a night of special favors, when prayers have a thousand times more virtue, lights are seen in the heavens, and water is said to become sweet."[10]

On this night, the Jandalis—and Muslims worldwide—are hoping to catch sight of the moon's first thin crescent that appears after sunset. For it will signal that the Islamic holy month of Ramadan has ended and that they may break their month-long fast.

After sighting the first new moon, Jandali and her family will now enjoy a meal as part of a festive repast that is eaten during daylight hours. Called the Feast of Breaking Fast *(Iд-al-Fitr)*, it is one of the great Muslim holidays. To express the specialness of the transition into the Feast of Breaking Fast, a Muslim writer shares this memory: "My father would take us to join the neighbors on some open field and relatively high ground shortly after sunset. We focused on the ... horizon, our hearts full of excitement and hope, to see the crescent that would herald the day of...eating delicious food after having fasted every day for the whole month."[11]

But before feasting, devout Muslims are asked to donate money to the poor and needy. By doing so, they can better recall the reason they fasted, and what it feels like to go without food and other comforts. For the deprivation and fasting done during Ramadan to be accepted by Allah, the charity must be donated *prior* to the prayer of thanks *(Salat)*.

During this time, cards and gifts are exchanged. Surrounded by family and friends, bathed in the *Qur'an*'s scripture and prayer to *Allah*, enjoying food that follows Islam's dietary guidelines—and that is eaten based on *adab* (manners) delineated in the *Qur'an* and the *Hadith*—the Feast of Breaking Fast has truly begun.

Islam's Essential Ingredients

To all appearances, Jandali and her family are simply breaking the daily fast of Ramadan, or are breaking the month-long fast with a feast on *Id-al-Fitr*. Yet beneath the surface celebration lies a fourteen-hundred-year-old tradition of forbidden foods and encouraged manners that are woven throughout the *Qur'an*. Islam is a religion that permeates all aspects of secular life—including what and how we eat. Whether avoiding pork, reaching for food that is closest to where you are sitting at the table, sitting while eating, chewing slowly and savoring the taste, not eating too many different types of food at any one meal, dining with others while framed in a feeling of kinship, or saying a prayer of appreciation both before and after eating—there is a devotional context for the food, and the social interaction that surrounds it.

"It is in the *Qur'an* that food is recognized as sustenance that is given to us through God," says Professor Algar. "Food has a dignity that deserves respect as a divine gift, a divine bounty." Indeed, the *Qur'an* professes that "all activities that sustain life should be undertaken with some degree of this awareness," he says.

Revered as the exact words that were revealed by God through the Angel Gabriel to the Prophet Muhammad over a period of twenty-three years, not a single word in the 114 chapters of the *Qur'an* has been changed during the last fourteen centuries. With a focus on all aspects of life that concern human beings, including food and eating, its basic tenet says that the relationship between God and all that He has created—from human beings, plants, and food, to animals, the earth, and the planet itself—is to be remembered, revered, and respected as God's creations.

One way in which the divine Law of the *Qur'an* encourages Muslims' submission to Allah is through the Five Pillars of Islam, the framework of Muslim life. The Five Pillars are: the declaration of faith *(Shahada)* which states that there is no god except God, and that Muhammad (a human being like ourselves) is His messenger; prayer *(Salat)*, which is performed five times daily as a direct link with God; fasting during Ramadan as a method of self-purification and a reminder to appreciate God's bounty; *Hajj*, a pilgrimage to the holy city of Mecca (Muhammad's birthplace) that should be done at least once during a person's lifetime, if health and finances permit; and *Zakat*, or charity, the underlying principle that all things belong to God, that 2.5 percent of one's income should be shared with those in need, and that the bounties we enjoy—including food—are treasures from Allah that we hold in trust.

Because Muslims believe the contents of the *Qur'an* came directly from Allah the Almighty God through Muhammad, and all the other great prophets before him (Moses, Jesus, etc.), "they never eat without first honoring the name of Allah," explains Dr. Sakr. "We eat in order to build up our body to stay as physically fit as possible. We do this so that we may utilize our body and our mind in the right way for the love of God, as well as for the sake of humankind."

Honoring Allah's Dietary Wisdom

Throughout the *Qur'an,* chapters remind Muslims that God created varieties of food on this earth to sustain humans. Therefore, people should never cause any harm to the face of the earth, or to the food God has provided.

Says Ameena Jandali: "Many Muslims may not realize that Islam is a highly environmental religion. It tells us that how we treat both our own bodies and the planet are serious responsibilities. This means that when we add anything artificial to our food—such as pesticides— we are disturbing God's plan." Writes Dr. Sakr, who is also a nutritionist: "Muslims are supposed to make an effort to obtain food of the best quality nutritionally (Qur'an 18:19)."[12]

Jandali concurs. "God created fruits, vegetables, and animals with wisdom," she says. "And by tampering with this wisdom — such as by putting chickens in cages and turning the lights on and off to make them produce more eggs, or by feeding cows hormones so that they will produce more milk — we disturb God's gift. Somewhere down the road, such disrespect is going to come back to haunt us."

Professor Algar echoes the same considerations: "To treat food in a disrespectful fashion is ultimately disrespectful to the *Qur'an* ... which tells us that food is sustenance that has been provided for us by *Allah*. Fast food, for instance, is the spiritual antithesis [of the dietary tenets of the *Qur'an*]." This means that by "treating food as an industrial artifact that is consumed without any devotional context" is to negate that food is a divine gift.

Indeed, the *Hadith*, Islam's prophetic traditions, tell us that the diet of the Prophet was very simple. His mainstays were fruits, vegetables, grains (especially barley), legumes, nuts, and seeds. The milk he drank was fresh and unprocessed, as were the eggs in his diet. "Because he lived simply," says Jandali, "lamb and other meat were not a mainstay."

Islam's "Mystical Menu"

In essence, the dietary wisdom of the *Qur'an* supports eating fresh foods in their natural state as often as possible. Because Islam says that we are responsible for our own bodies and the earth that is a divine gift, anything that may be harmful to the body or planet should be avoided.

The *Qur'an* also tells us that God bestowed His blessings *(barakah)* on Humankind by creating a Divine bounty of food that is to be honored and enjoyed. To solidify and clarify this holy relationship to food, the *Qur'an* is resplendent with dietary laws and guidelines. But the Muslim relationship to food goes deeper than the mere words and ritual of the dietary codes, for "we are also asked to concentrate our minds, hearts, and spirits on the pleasure of Allah when we eat," says Dr. Sakr. The will of Allah, the divine God, and the blessings inherent in food, stand at the center of all dining endeavors.

Nowhere is this profound relationship more evident than in *Sufism,* the mystical strain of Islam to which some devotees have turned in order to attain higher levels of spiritual fulfillment.[13] Found throughout Islamic communities worldwide, those choosing the Sufi Path follow beliefs that are closely linked to the *Qur'an,* but Sufis also seek direct union with God.

Neither a sect nor school of thought, Sufism "is rather a spiritual or transcendental practice. . . . [Sufis] seek a life of ascetic pietism . . . and the inward purity of a relationship with God through love, patience, forgiveness, and other higher spiritual qualities,"[14] explains M. Cherif Bassiouni.

Perhaps nowhere is the pursuit of "higher spiritual qualities" more evident than in Sufis' relationship to food. In fact, Professor Algar told me, novices in Sufi orders train in the kitchen "not because it is menial," but because Sufis believe that "in the preparation of the food is the maturing of the human soul." In the realm of Sufism, "Sufis would not eat food prepared by someone who had not been in a state of ritual purity while cooking," he notes. "From the point of view of Sufis, that lack of purity is transferred into the food."

Ayla Algar, Professor Algar's wife and a lecturer in Turkish language and literature at the University of California, Berkeley, explains in her writings about Sufi beliefs that for Turkish Sufis, food is lush with spiritual symbolism and sustenance. Algar quotes what writer Anne-Marie Schimmel calls the "mystical menu" integrated throughout some of Turkish poet Mevlana's (better known in the West as Rumi) poetry about Sufis;[15] it is poetry that infuses food with profound divine meaning.

Writes Ayla Algar about this poetry: "Wholesome food corresponds to spiritual nourishment, and its cooking and preparation parallel the refinement and advancement of the soul. The relation of body to soul is like that of sour milk to butter; only after separation from the milk does the butter become tasty and distinct, and the soul likewise attains its perfection through gradual separation from the body.... *Helva* [a sweet made from sesame seeds] is perhaps Mevlana's favorite among foods," posits Algar, "for its sweetness has affinity to the sweetness of spiritual experience:"[16] Once spiritual pleasures are tasted, those of the world are spurned.

Islam's Spiritual Sustenance

A memorable story told to me by Ameena Jandali reflects Islam's sacred relationship to food: "When I lived in Turkey," she told me, "I would often see walls upon which were pieces of bread. Muslims had placed them there because bread is considered to be God's bounty. Therefore, it is considered improper, sacrilegious, for food to be on the floor where it could be stepped on. For if you step on food, you are stepping on God's bounty, Allah's gift to us."

At its core, "Islam's dietary wisdom tells us that food is divine in its origin, and that Allah provided it for us as sustenance for our beings," says Professor Algar. "It tells us that food deserves our respect and veneration at all times. For food has come to us through God; it is the material of Allah."

Indeed, eating is a sacred act, an opportunity to partake of "the material of Allah." And as we do, we experience *barakah*, the blessing from God that is food.

Devout Dietary Wisdom

What exactly are the dietary codes in the *Qur'an* that inspire such sweet spiritual inspiration? They are two-dimensional: one aspect of the dietary code includes laws that specify forbidden foods and, as in Judaism, compassionate ways in which to slaughter food animals; the other focus encourages particular manners *(adab)* and food-related behavior designed to enhance a God-consciousness *(Taqwa)*. Whether they are dietary laws or etiquette guidelines, all are designed to encourage Muslims to remember always that "eating is considered to be a matter of worship of God."[17]

What follows is an overview of Islam's dietary code gleaned from the *Qur'an*. Much of the content was synthesized and explained to me by Dr. Sakr,[18] former professor and chairman of the Department of Chemistry and Nutrition at the National College of Chiropractic in Lombard, Illinois, and founder of the Foundation for Islamic Knowledge in Walnut, California. In the spirit of Islam, consider viewing the laws and guidelines through the lens of *Ihsan,* the highest level of faith that encourages devout Muslims to behave in their daily life as if God is present at all times and in all things—including in the food on their plates.

Lawful (Halal):

Compassionately slaughtered animals. Only animals that have been properly slaughtered are edible. This includes saying the name of God before shooting an animal, or cutting the animal's throat, because it is considered the most merciful way of taking an animal's life. Believed to contain impurities that may harm the body, all blood must be drained from the animal's body. Only meat slaughtered by those who have received a divine scripture—Muslims, Jews, and Christians—is considered acceptable.

Edible flesh. Meat, birds, fish, and foul are considered lawful, unless specifically declared unlawful. All seafood and fish are acceptable, but Muslims believe that the meat one eats should only be slaughtered in God's name, which gives, it an inherent dignity that deserves respect. Animals that have been deemed edible may only be slaughtered for human sustenance.

Dairy. The consumption of unadulterated milk products (cheese, milk, butter, etc.) is encouraged; all dairy products, including eggs, are lawful.

Plant-based food. Plants are harvested for our survival. To keep the body healthy, the consumption of fresh, whole food in its natural state is encouraged. Plant-based foods were also the staple for Muhammad the Prophet. These include fruits, vegetables, grains, beans and peas, nuts, and seeds.

Other. Pure honey, mentioned throughout the *Qur'an*, is highly recommended, as are dates and vegetable oil, especially olive oil. When presented with a new, unfamiliar food, a Muslim is asked to become aware of the ingredients before eating it.

Unlawful (Haram):

"Non-divine" slaughtering *(Zabiha).* Meat of animals slaughtered by atheists is considered unlawful; so is meat that has been slaughtered by anyone who has not received a divine scripture, or who has dedicated the animal to any other than God.

Certain flesh. Because pigs are considered unclean, pork and other food products from swine are forbidden. Other unclean animals include birds of prey, crawling insects and animals, dogs, asses, and mules.

"Non-compassionate" deaths. The manner in which an animal died also determines whether it is edible. For instance, forbidden for consumption are animals that have died violently, such as through strangulation, a fall, or a violent blow; or an animal or bird that has been partially devoured (perhaps by a wild animal). Even if an animal is legal, it is unlawful to consume it if it has not been slaughtered in an acceptable, compassionate manner.

Intoxicating liquids. All liquids are acceptable, except those that are capable of causing intoxication. Therefore, Islam prohibits the consumption of alcohol. The reason: intoxicants are harmful to the body; they are also potentially harmful (indirectly) to those who come into contact with the intoxicated person. The main purpose for avoidance, though, is that being inebriated keeps us from being God-conscious at all times.

Questionable Foods:

"Suspected" food. If a Muslim is presented with a food or drink that is not clearly legal or prohibited, she or he is asked to make a personal judgment call about whether to eat the food. Such "in between" food is considered questionable *(Shubba)*. Practicing Muslims are discouraged from putting themselves in a position where they must decide if food is "suspected." This applies to any food or diet that is not specifically recommended.

"Discouraged" food. Any food, drink, or drugs that may harm a person's health *(Makrooh)* are religiously discouraged — even detested. If a person consumes *Makrooh* products knowingly, he or she may be "blamed" on the Day of Judgment. Some examples include drugs (such as stimulants and depressants), cigarette smoke, and stimulants (including caffeine-containing beverages such as coffee, tea, and soft drinks).

Recommended Etiquette:

Wash before eating. Washing your hands and other extremities before eating is recommended, for it is a sign of ritual purity. It is both a literal and symbolic gesture: while dining, not only should the body be clean, so too should the mind and heart.

Be God-conscious. Because God created food for us, it is considered sacred. Therefore, eat in the name of God, and finish meals by thanking God for making the food available to you. Be grateful to God, and appreciate and show respect for the divine gift of food.

Pray devoutly. Thank Allah before and after eating. In addition to prayers said before and after mealtime, Muslims pray five times daily. Their prayers include much movement: bowing forward, standing up, and full prostrations on the floor. All this movement enhances digestion.

In the name of God, we harvest the food
In the name of God, we eat it
In the name of God, we distribute it.

Do not abuse food. Because food is a gift from God, it is sinful to abuse it. To honor our body and God's bounty, the *Qur'an* suggests eating the best of what is on this planet—and eating neither too much nor too little. Therefore, strive to eat the amount of food your body needs to keep it healthy.

Avoid wasting food. In the *Qur'an*, we are considered sinners if we throw out or waste any food. This means that extra food should be put in the refrigerator to be eaten later. We also have no right to take the life of an animal for food and then not eat its flesh.

Eat with others. Islam is a social religion. It encourages Muslims to dine with family, friends, and neighbors, for the blessing is with the company. By eating together in the name of God, we may feel truly nourished. Also, the strength and coherence of the family as a unit is manifested when you're eating together. Islam goes so far as to suggest that the aroma of food that is being cooked should encourage neighbors to come by and share in the meal. In this way, members of society are brought together in the name of Allah.

Share food with others. Because both food and human beings are sacred, food is to be shared with others who are less fortunate or hungry. The *Qur'an* suggests giving part of what you eat to other people, or to hungry animals. By feeding others who are hungry, you share in the reward.

Select "nearby" food. When Muslims dine together in large groups, food is often served in one large pot or on a very large platter (perhaps four feet in diameter). It is considered polite to serve yourself by selecting a portion of food that is closest to you on the platter. The reason: it is a blessing to eat as one big family.

Eat simply. The fewer types of food—or dishes—that are eaten together at any one meal, the better. This encourages satisfaction with simple foods, as well as easy digestion. By not impressing others with fancy, expensive, or elaborate food or dishes, it also encourages humbleness.

Do not overeat. Avoid eating to the point of satiety and satisfaction. For optimal digestion, the stomach should be filled one-third with food solids, one-third with liquid from the food, and one-third left empty. Stopping before feeling full brings peace of mind, because we do not abuse what God has given to us while others go hungry.

Chew and drink slowly. Eating food quickly or gulping down liquids, without conscious, reverential recognition of the nourishment, is to treat food—and therefore, the *Qur'an* and God—in a disrespectful fashion. Chewing slowly, with awareness, represents a conscious understanding that the food is being provided by God.

Sit down when eating. Being seated and focusing on food and liquids while eating or drinking reinforces respect for the sustenance God has provided.

Eat three times daily. Eat only when you feel hungry. In the Middle East, lunch is the largest, heaviest meal; the evening meal is the lightest, so that it will not disturb sleep.

Consume liquids between meals. Muslims are encouraged to consume liquids perhaps an hour or two after food has been eaten. Keeping liquids separate from foodstuff is believed to enhance digestion.

Rest after eating. If possible, relax after eating. Rest quietly for about fifteen minutes to give the food time to digest properly. If you start to work, or begin physical activity shortly after eating, blood will be diverted to the circulatory system, and the stomach may not receive sufficient blood for optimal digestion.

Fast occasionally. Abstaining from food is seen as an opportunity to purify both body and mind, improve health, and to live calmly and peacefully. Through fasting, we develop a keener appreciation of the bounty of food that God has given us. It reminds us of our dependence on food, and helps us to realize there are many whose hunger is not voluntary. While fasting, provide food for the poor and hungry. In addition to the month of Ramadan, Islam encourages Muslims to fast on Mondays and Thursdays and on six days in the month of *Shawwal* (the month following Ramadan).

seven

Buddhism: Mindful Meals

The great Master Dogen taught: The practice of
eating is the essential truth of all dharmas (the teachings of Buddhism and universal truth). At the very
moment of eating, we merge with ultimate reality.
Thus dharma is eating, and eating is dharma. And
this eating is full of holy joy and ecstasy.[1]

—*Abbot John Daido Loori*

When Siddhartha Gautama realized his true essence while sitting under a Bodhi Tree in Northern India 2,500 years ago, thus
becoming the **Buddha,** he set forth a spiritual philosophy, a moral and
ethical practice, that includes showing how to transform everyday
experiences, such as eating, into sacred activity that is capable of
revealing our true nature. Buddhism maintains that **enlightenment**—
an awakening beyond word and thought—is our natural state, one
that may be experienced by bringing a mindful, meditative awareness
to all aspects of our lives, including food: its selection, preparation,
serving, the act of eating itself, even the "clean-up" and metabolism
that occurs after we've eaten. What follows is a visit into the similar-
yet-different culinary consciousnesses of two Buddhist-influenced
cultures—Japan and Tibet: Japan's Zen Buddhist monastic mindful
food meditations, and Tibet's Tantric Buddhist consciousness that
transforms food into sacred art. Such practices are designed to free
our inner wisdom and reveal the true, resplendent non-self self.

Minding the Monastic Meal

It is meal time at the Zen Mountain Monastery in Mt. Tremper, New York. Forty-five retreatants are participating in *Oryoki*[2]—a formal monastery meal served during intense periods of training. The ceremony is rich with silence, the "container" that allows the spiritual work to be done.

To begin, each person picks up his or her personal bowls and utensils wrapped in cloth from shelves at the entrance of the meditation hall. Maintaining silence, they walk toward their sitting mats holding their bowls at eye level. By doing so, they are expressing gratitude and identification with the spiritual largess of the Buddha. Once they each have a set of bowls and utensils, they remain standing at their mats until a clapper is struck, signaling that it is time to be seated.

When the food is ready to be served, a meal bell is struck five times. Then a thundering drum roll permeates the hall as a priest and cook (who does the liturgy) enter to present the food as an offering to Buddha at the main altar. As the two exit, all the retreatants recite a chant that initiates the beginning of the meal. Then, everybody unwraps the three "nested" bowls, utensils, and place mat that are wrapped in the knotted cloths, setting them out in a precise, detailed procedure—all at the same time—until a complete place setting is arranged before each person.

After this process, the *Ino* (head of the meditation room) strikes a gavel on a flat, thick, wooden block; then the chanting of the names of various Buddhas commences. At the same time, servers enter the hall with the meal's condiments, serving them to the seated retreatants on small trays.

Shortly afterward, other servers follow suit with the food for the Buddha bowl, the largest round bowl of the three at each place setting, as well as food for the other two bowls. For this particular meal, rice is served into the Buddha bowl; the second, medium-size bowl holds a bean dish; and the third, smallest bowl is held out to the servers so that it may be filled with a medley of baked vegetables. To indicate to the servers when the exact, correct amount of each food has been received, each person gestures slightly upward with palm upturned.

The chanting of the Buddhas' names continues throughout the serving process, as does the use of other hand gestures. For instance, placing the thumb and forefinger together indicates the wish for a small portion of food. Also ongoing is *zazen*, the Japanese Zen Buddhist term for mindful, sitting meditation. Indeed, the word *Zen* is derived from the word *dhyana*, the Sanskrit word meaning meditation.

After everyone has been served, the pre-meal chant commences. It is recited as specific *mudras* (symbolic hand gestures) are made, which change throughout the chant:[3]

> *First, seventy-two labors brought us this food;*[4]
> *We should know how it comes to us.*[5]
> *Second, as we receive this offering,*
> *We should consider*
> *Whether our virtue and practice deserve it.*
> *Third, as we desire the natural order of mind*
> *To be free from clinging,*
> *We must be free from greed.*
> *Fourth, to support our life we take this food.*
> *Fifth, to attain our way we take this food.*[6]
>
> *First, this food is for the Three Treasures.*
> *Second, it is for our teachers,*[7] *parents, nation,*
> *And all sentient beings.*
> *Third, it is for all beings in the six worlds.*[8]
> *Thus, we eat this food with everyone.*
> *We eat to stop all evil, to practice good,*
> *To save all sentient beings,*
> *And to accomplish our Buddha Way.*[9]

As everybody eats, servers collect a food offering, a "pinch" of food that each eater has left on the utensil;[10] they also gather up the condiments. As each person completes the meal, he or she resumes meditation, until all have finished the meal and all are meditating.

Leaving No Traces

It is now that the *Ino* signals the beginning of the intricate clean-up procedure. The *Ino* starts by cleaning both the spoon and chopsticks with the tongue (while a hand is covering the mouth). Next, using a small cleaning stick, the *Ino* cleans all residual food from all three bowls. The same cleaning process is followed by everybody.

The next stage of the clean-up, washing the bowls, begins when hot tea is served into each retreatant's Buddha bowl. Using the spatula to swirl the water around, each person proceeds to clean all traces of food in the Buddha bowl. When no more traces of food remain, they transfer the water into the next-smaller bowls. Before proceeding to clean it with the water, each participant first dries the Buddha bowl, and washes, cleans, and dries the utensils, then places them inside the utensil bag.

The cleaning process is repeated until the remaining two bowls have been washed and wiped dry with a cloth. Then the spatula (which has been used as the cleaning tool) is cleaned, dried, and returned to the utensil bag. With the nested bowls and utensils clean and in place, each person either takes a sip or drinks all of the remaining water. Then, still sitting with hands placed in the *gassho* (acknowledgment) *mudra*, palms together in front of their faces, servers collect any residual, unused water. During this stage, the "muddy water" chant is recited by all:

> *The water with which I wash these bowls*
> *Tastes like ambrosia;*
> *I offer it to the various spirits to satisfy them.*[11]

Now the remaining bowl is washed and dried, returned to its nesting order, and retied with a simple knot in the cloth. As each person finishes this stage of the procedure, he or she returns to *zazen* meditation. Then, when all are practicing sitting meditation, the *Ino* chants:

> *May we exist in muddy water with purity like a lotus.*
> *Thus we bow to Buddha.*[12]

Next, after a slight bow, the wrapped-up dining paraphernalia is brought to the forehead in a brief gesture. Keeping the bowls at eye level, everyone stands, preparing to leave the meditation hall.

A bell rings, the drum rolls, there is bowing to the right, a bell rings, there is another bow to the left, then all the retreatants bow to each other. Again the bell rings as the pace of the drum quickens. Everyone stands in place, still holding the bowls at eye level.

When the drum stops abruptly and the bell rings, the participants begin their procession out of the meditation hall, returning the wrapped-up bowls and utensils to the shelves just outside the hall. The meal is officially over—with no remaining traces of food or waste.[13] What is left is the experience that stays in the hearts and minds of those who participated in the meal.

The Buddha in Food

With its many details, motions, and movements, it may be easy to perceive the *Oryoki* meal as a prescribed religious ritual. But within the practice of Buddhism, monastic meals—indeed, all meals and other "everyday" activities—serve as a microcosm for the more profound, all-encompassing essence of Buddhism. The formal *Oryoki* monastery meal "is a state of mind, not a ritual,"[14] explains Abbot John Daido Loori of the Zen Mountain Monastery. Daido Loori is an ordained Buddhist priest and teacher who has received transmission (sanctioned acknowledgment from a teacher of achievement of the realized state) in the Soto and Rinzai Zen Buddhist lineages.

And what is this "state of mind?" Says Daido Loori: "If Dharma [the spiritual essence and teachings of Buddhism] is the Dharma nature, a meal also is the Dharma nature.... If Dharma is one mind, a meal is also one mind.... If Dharma is enlightenment, then food is enlightenment."[15]

For Buddhists, the state of enlightenment is a major motivation for practicing intense mindful meditation during all "everyday" activities, including each meal. Through such concentrated absorption, practicing Buddhists become aware of the moment-to-moment quality of life and, potentially, the inherent temporariness and impermanence of thoughts, feelings, and things. In turn, through such detachment, comes the ability to see the transitory nature of experiences and the veil of false perceptions and social conditioning is lifted. In its place is *enlightenment*, the experience of seeing people, situations, and objects — in other words, life — in a state of full awareness and consciousness.

Ingredients of Buddhism

The practice and cultivation of mindful awareness meditation is rooted in one of Buddhism's earliest *sutras*, ancient Buddhist teachings. Called the *Mindfulness Sutra*, "it is a description of how to cultivate mindfulness of the body, feelings, thoughts," and ultimately, "mindful awareness in every moment," explains Yvonne Rand, a meditation teacher and priest in the Zen tradition.[16] Basically, "it is an awareness that is free of judgment, that is impartial and 'awake' to what is going on in the moment — to the situation, the detail of what you are doing."

Mindfulness meditation evolved from Buddha's Noble Eightfold Path which, tradition says, he presented more than two thousand five hundred years ago after his enlightenment during a discourse on the turning of the Wheel of Dharma. The Eightfold Path includes right view, right thought, right speech, right conduct, right livelihood, right effort, right mindfulness, and right meditation.

In turn, the Eightfold Path is based in the Buddha's core Four Noble Truths: the fact of suffering (birth, aging, illness, dying); its causes (cravings, reincarnation, passion for pleasure); its cessation (ceasing attachment to cravings, and releasing fears of abandonment, rejection, etc.); and the path to the cessation of suffering, which includes mindfulness meditation and the other elements of the Noble Eightfold Path.[17]

Bringing Mindfulness to Meals

Based on Buddha's meditative experience and ensuing enlightenment, bringing a meditative awareness to food is seen as one way to attain this essential truth; the practice of mindfulness takes precedence over the food itself which, in Zen Buddhism, is usually vegetarian. Although meat is not explicitly forbidden in all Buddhist traditions, a vow against killing is interpreted by many to include avoiding the ingestion of animal flesh.[18]

For some devout Buddhists, both plant- and animal-based food are considered to be sentient beings; therefore, no matter what is eaten, the belief is that a life is being taken so that human beings may have energy to live. Such an awareness makes the *Oryoki* meal an especially profound ritual, for the mindfulness inherent in it is an expression of appreciation and gratitude—an acknowledgment that something died so that human beings may live. Such awareness is transformed into spiritual work, the practice of enlightenment.

Believing that all beings are Buddha nature, Dogen Kigen, the thirteenth-century founder of the Soto Zen school in Japan, emphasized that enlightenment was not something only *potentially* to be realized, but was an *actuality* that could be manifested in the "here and now" through ongoing sitting meditation.[19] Realizing the role food could play in both being in, and achieving the enlightened state, Master Dogen developed the monastic meal meditation and, as Abbot Loori explains, "made the position of chief cook...one of the most important ones at the monastery—usually second only to the Abbot." Even now, it is a teaching position that receives much respect and regard.

Some would say that the process of eating itself is a "teacher," pregnant with enlightening possibilities. Explains Yvonne Rand: "There is a whole way of eating in Zen that comes out of the meditation tradition." Ultimately, "how Buddhists eat and what we eat is an expression of spiritual life. It is about the cultivation of mindful awareness in eating."

I spoke with Rand on the grounds of her extraordinary home, which is also a retreat center, located near the Pacific Ocean in a small community north of San Francisco. As we talked in an enclosed gazebo-like room, she wore a maroon-colored robe "that was given to me by one of my teachers who is a Tibetan lama," she explained. Stitched in the pattern of a rice paddy, "it symbolizes that one takes refuge in the Buddha."

It is possible to "take refuge in the Buddha" each time we eat mindfully. For instance, according to Rand, cultivating mindfulness in eating may include: awareness of the pace at which you eat; the attention you give to the physical detail of eating; sensing the texture and flavor of the food in your mouth, including swallowing; cultivating awareness of every detail in the act of eating; being mindful of how you handle your utensils and bowls when eating; and also of your posture while you eat, such as keeping your back straight. "When your back is straight, you are the most alert," Rand explains.

Tibet's "Buttery" Buddha Offerings

It is midnight in the holy city of Lhasa, Tibet. The thermometer hovers around ten degrees as the crowd of Tibetan Buddhist laypeople and monastics celebrate the New Year (Lo-gsar). During the last few hours, the crowd has swelled to more than a million, all wishing to pray close to the massive hand-molded butter sculptures (tormas) that surround a sacred statue of the Buddha. As the new year begins, they are praying for the exorcism of negative influences and requesting good fortune for the coming year.

Each butter sculpture is perhaps sixty feet high—as high as a two- or three-story house. There may be fifty or sixty of these huge sculptures surrounding the Jokhang, or cathedral. Within the Jokhang is a large statue of the Buddha that is believed to have been made around the time Buddha achieved enlightenment.

The maroon-robed monks (the color represents their connection to the earth and nonmaterialism) who create the gigantic sculptures begin to make the sculptures two to three weeks before the new year. Thousands of monks are involved in their creation, working day and night for three weeks. So that the monastics are able to create the sacred butter sculptures, "living Buddhas and affluent patrons of the monastery had contributed... nearly thirteen thousand pounds of yak butter," notes writer Joseph R. Rock.[20]

While creating the sculptures, the mindfulness of the monks is intense. Says Lama Kunga Rinpoche, who learned to create the butter sculptures in his homeland of Tibet: "While we are making the butter sculptures, our mindfulness is very strong. We are taught to be artists and think about nothing else; no daydreaming. Your mind flows with your fingers, the hours pass... and we do the job."[21]

To create the sacred butter sculptures, the monks pinch off pieces of yak butter (made from the *dri,* a female yak), dip them into a bowl of iced water so the butter will hold its shape, and gracefully sculpt whatever image they choose by pasting the small bits of pre-colored butter — piece by piece — on plywood forms that have been carved into the desired shape. Images range from the Buddha and famous saints and sages to flowers, dragons, and mandalas described by Tibetan Lama Yeshe as "circular diagram[s] symbolic of the entire universe."[22]

Consider these descriptions of butter sculptures created by Tibetan monks, reported by a writer for *National Geographic* magazine in 1928, well before China, under the aegis of its Cultural Revolution, destroyed most of Tibet's monasteries and, along with them, monastic life and many of its spiritual ceremonies:[23]

- The fierce Gombo is the most venerated deity in Tibet. Here the butter sculptor depicts him in the pit of fire, treading underfoot the elephant-headed god Ganesha, his son.

- This exquisite figure is Donker, one of the twenty-one manifestations of Drolma, the Goddess of Mercy.

- This masterpiece of butter sculpture is a monk's conception of the patron saint of Lhasa, the deity to whom alone a Tibetan prayer is addressed.

To learn more about the art and spiritual essence behind the creation of the butter sculptures, I spoke with Tibetan Lama Kunga Rinpoche of the Ewam Choden Center, a Tibetan Buddhist meditation center in Kensington, California.[24] Born in 1935 in Tibet, Rinpoche lived there for almost twenty-five years, learning the sacred art of butter sculpting while studying at the Ngor Monastery, which was built in the 1400s. After his father was imprisoned by the Chinese and the monastery destroyed, he moved to the United States in 1962. Permitted to return to Tibet in 1979, he brought his father back to the United States in 1980. This is what he told me about a typical butter festival:

"Surrounding the butter sculptures are offerings for the five senses: butter lamps (for sight offerings); perfumes (smell offerings); the *torma* (cake made with butter and sugar) as a taste offering; flowers (touch offerings); and music played by the monks, especially cymbals (as hearing offerings). The senses are important to the human being. By filling the senses with these things, we're hoping to be filled with love and a sense of beauty.

"The butter lamps, which contain yak butter that is melted and purified, are filled with wicks. The monks line up the butter lamps on the banks that surround the butter sculptures, then light them so that the sculptures can be seen. The sculptures represent something to eat. And the *ghee* (purified or clarified butter) from the butter makes a flame of light, which represents enlightenment. It's the middle of the night and many monks are sitting, looking toward the sculptures, and they are praying:

> *May all sentient beings be happy.*
> *May all sentient beings be free from suffering, and the sources*
> *of suffering.*
> *May all become enlightened by the offering of the sculpture*
> *and the butter lamps to Buddha.*

"The butter sculptures are left outside for one night only, during which time about a million people walk around the sculptures and say prayers for themselves and others. The next morning the monks dismount the butter sculptures and give them to the birds and dogs. They give them to the beggars and homeless people, who eat the butter."

"Buttery" Buddhist Beliefs

To grasp the significance of the butter sculptures is to appreciate that their creation is a form of visualization meditation created in the fifteenth century by the scholar monk Je Tsong Khapa. As with other meditation practices, it is designed to lift the veil of illusion and illuminate the "Buddha consciousness" that cannot be grasped with the rational mind.

The creation of these *torma* offerings (also called *martor; mar* means "butter," *tor* means "sculpture") is a meditation practice specific to Tibetan Buddhism, alternately called Tantra, "esoteric," or "mystical" Buddhism. Created as part of the Mahayana Buddhist tradition in the third century C.E., the Tantric tradition embraces the "eighty-four thousand" *sutra* teachings of the Buddha and the "three jewels," meaning the Buddha (enlightenment), the dharma (teachings), and the *sangha* (the enlightened community).

Basically, says writer Linda Johnsen, "for tantrics, tantra means uncovering the undying reality within ourselves through meditation, yoga, ritual, selfless service, art, study, self-inquiry, and especially devotion to the divine in whatever form they conceive of Her."[25]

Tibetan tantrics also use the principles of mind turnings—one of the Tantric paths to enlightenment—to travel on what Buddhist nun Carol Corradi explains as the Tibetan "graduated path to enlightenment."[26] I talked with Carol Corradi, director of the Tse Chen Ling Center in San Francisco, about the butter sculptures, Tibetan Buddhism, and mind turnings during a conversation in a local cafe. Each word she spoke reflected her authenticity, intelligence, and passion for her practice.

In essence, she said, the turnings include: the preciousness of human rebirth (reincarnation); appreciating the relevance of *karma* (the concept of cause and effect—that we are responsible for our actions); understanding the emptiness of human life ("the absence of false ideas about how things exist");[27] the realization of death (seen as "the separation of the mind from the body at the end of one's life");[28] the reliance on a lama ("a spiritual guide or teacher in the Buddhist traditions of Tibet");[29] and the recognition of impermanence, that all phenomena is transitory and impermanent.

To remember the transitory, impermanent nature of all things, the material used to make the sculptures is purposefully impermanent. Explains Lama Kunga Rinpoche: "Butter from the female yak...comes from high up in the mountains. It is rare and considered to be a pure essence from the earth. In the Buddhist tradition, whatever is the rarest, the most precious, is the first thing that is offered to God, the Buddha. This is why we create the butter sculptures."

But, Lama Kunga Rinpoche explained, *tormas*, when not used for the New Year ceremony, can also be sculpted by combining flour, butter, sugar, and water and made into cakes to be offered to Buddha. You can bake them and, when they're done, put them on a plate, then place them in front of an altar as an offering to Buddha.

"Everything is impermanent," he continues. "The sculptures are beautiful and then they're gone—as are our lives. It is important to remember the impermanence of life, because with attachment (to life—or anything) comes suffering. By learning detachment, you can enjoy something when you have it; when you don't, and it's gone, just let it be."

Yvonne Rand concurs. Creating the full sculpture and then dissolving it "is the quintessential reminder that one of the marks of everything that comes into existence is that it will pass out of existence. This is one of the core focuses in Buddhism."

Adds Carol Corradi: "When I make cake *tormas*, I'm taking food that is part of my life, part of the ordinary, and making it into something more. By elevating the food, I elevate my own self and make that connection with the enlightened nature. It brings me out of the ordinary."

As with the Zen monastic meal, after the sculptures are dismantled and "recycled" as a gift to others or nature (or eaten, if they are in the form of sculpted pastries), no traces remain. And, just as Zen monastics offer a pinch of food to the Buddha as an offering during a meal, so, too, do the monks of Tibet use butter to create an offering to the Buddha in the form of sacred art. And, as with all food, "the butter sculptures are offerings to enlightened, holy beings, as well as the enlightened nature within ourselves...our Buddha potential," explains Corradi.

Partaking of the Nectar

Abbot John Daido Loori tells the story of a cook in Nelson, New Zealand, who once prepared the meals during an intensive meditation retreat. "Most of you know how I feel about modern vegetarian food," he says. "It seems bland and lacking any vitality. [But] this guy's cooking is absolutely exquisite, the tastiest vegetarian cooking I've ever had in my life."[30]

The secret? The way the cook regarded the food. "He handles those cabbage leaves as if they were his children," says Daido Loori. "He handles them with loving kindness, with intimacy, with joy, and with a profound respect." By preparing food with "wisdom, compassion, love—we *eat* [emphasis added] wisdom, compassion, love," he says. "It nourishes us, we in turn nourish each other and return it to ...whence it came."

Buddhism's mindfulness and visualization meditations suggest that each time we eat—or even look at food—we have an opportunity to create and experience the Buddha consciousness inherent in both food and ourselves. But "the extent to which our food reveals itself depends on us," writes Thich Nhat Hanh, as well as our heartfelt ability to regard food with "wisdom, compassion, and love."[31]

It depends on your approaching each meal mindfully, with ongoing awareness. When you do, you are "in" the Buddha nature inherent in both yourself and food. And, as Carol Corradi says, in the process you are being nourished by "the nectar of which enlightened beings partake."

Practicing Mindful Meal Meditation

You don't have to make a butter sculpture or sit on a floor mat to practice mindful eating. Mindfulness may be used at any time, any meal, to transform an apparently ordinary meal into something extraordinary, something more than it is, "something of nectar" as Carol Corradi calls it. To enter this "state of being," she suggests beginning with a "mental offering," a recognition that before you eat, you're offering the food to an enlightened being, the Buddha, as well as to all enlightened beings.

Next, she suggests acknowledging that a transformation is taking place, that food is more than mundane, that it represents something you can use to recall the enlightened nature within yourself. "This visualization turns the food into the nectar that all enlightened beings partake of," she says. "It's a transubstantiation in the sense of making the food the embodiment of any entity. It's taking ourselves to a spiritual level—and our food with it."

To eat mindfully and "offer your best" is to live in the present. It calls for paying attention to every act, every sensation and perception, for its own sake, in the moment. It is to sense your senses and feel your feelings from a detached, observant viewpoint. Such is the state of awareness you bring to any phase of a meal.

Such a state is real rather than symbolic, meaning it is an experience that is located in sensations rather than abstractions. In the Buddhist worldview, for instance, an egg does not represent a microcosm of the world; rather, it simply is an oval-shaped item with certain characteristics.

To experience a meal with a mindful awareness, consider organizing a meal around its phases: planning, preparation, serving, eating, and clean-up. Regardless of which stage or stages of the meal on which you choose to focus, the important point is *not* to let your mind become distracted. This is because being mindful means that you are aware of an action while you're doing it—as well as after.

For instance, before you reach for a fork, acknowledge—consciously—that you intend to reach for the fork; then notice your hand reaching for it and picking it up; sense the fork as you hold it in your hand, and so on. The mindfulness is on whatever stage of meal preparation you're in. Focus on your intention, observe your actions and the effects of your actions. Consider that eating is action and sensation.

In essence, you're taking your actions off "automatic pilot" mode and, instead, are committed to being fully aware of what your hand, mouth, and mind are experiencing moment to moment. Your mind will slip away from the present. When you become aware that it has, simply and without judgment bring it back to the present moment. From the start to finish of your meal, your intention is to link the moments together into a continuous stream of sensory awareness. Try it and you will find out how difficult this can be.

Being mindful. To become focused, become silent and breathe in a relaxed manner. Choose a time when you're not hurried or distracted by other things. Avoid television, radio, books, or newspapers. Don't take phone calls. Instead, focus on maintaining a continuous moment-by-moment awareness throughout the whole meal-making/taking process: visualization, planning, preparing, serving, eating, cleaning up, and digestion.

Visualizing the meal. Become focused in your mind's eye on what you're going to prepare—its appearance, aroma, ingredients, etc. If other thoughts enter your mind, such as this will take too much time, give the thought your attention, then let it pass on so that you can bring yourself back to the meal visualization. Simply witness the thought until it passes on.

Planning the meal. Mentally focus on all the steps involved in preparing the meal. When will you prepare it? For whom will you prepare it? What will you make? Run through every phase of the planning process: What part of the meal or dish will you prepare first? Where will you buy the groceries? Which ingredients do you already have? If you go shopping for the food, be aware of each action you take as you push the grocery cart down the aisle. Focus on the actions you make as you select the foods.

Preparing the meal. Be mindful of the action of washing the food, such as vegetables you may be preparing for a fresh salad. Notice yourself reaching for the refrigerator door. Observe the other vegetables in the refrigerator. Acknowledge the action of reaching for the vegetables. Do the same with the meal's utensils, pots, and dishes as well as with the mixing, blending, and cooking of the dish.

Setting the table. The table on which you eat can be as sacred as the rest of the meal. Create a table that is inviting, for both you and the food. What are the colors and textures of the placemats or tablecloth? Are the utensils pleasing? Consider complementing the meal with a flower arrangement. Or light candles — even if it's breakfast time.

Serving the meal. Be mindful of each action associated with serving the meal: selecting dishes and utensils, setting the table, bringing the food to the table, etc. Reap the benefits of the visualization meditation of the Tibetan monks by presenting the food as if it were a sacred work of art. Notice the colors, the placement of the food on the plate. You're witnessing your mind noticing the food.

Eating the meal. As with the Zen monastic meal, be mindful of each aspect of the food you're eating. To begin, consider saying words of thanks or appreciation for the food. Savor the aroma of the food by inhaling deeply. Notice yourself reaching for the fork, selecting some food, placing the food in your mouth, removing the fork, placing it back on the plate as you chew the mouthful. Regard the motion of your hand and arm. Chew slowly, identifying the different levels of flavors that you taste. Experience the texture and taste sensations. Do you chew more on the right or left side of your mouth? When do you become ready to swallow? Observe each motion involved in the taking of the next mouthful of food.

Cleaning up. Regard this as a sacred process, too. It is just as important a part of the meal as the other phases. Resenting this stage takes you out of the moment of being. Vietnamese Zen master Thich Nhat Hanh says, "I know that if I hurry...the time of washing dishes will be unpleasant and not worth living. That would be a pity, for each minute, each second of life is a miracle. The dishes themselves and the fact that I am here washing them are miracles!"[31]

Digesting the food. After you've eaten, be aware of how the food feels in your stomach, how you're feeling. For instance, are you aware that you overate, are still hungry, or ate just the right amount? Witness the effects of having eaten the meal. For in the witnessing lies the essence of life itself.

eight

China and Japan: Food Folklore, Tea Treasure

Foods are used in...festivals as a way of communicating with gods, ghosts, and ancestors. Once the spirits consume the "essence" of the food, it is shared with friends and relatives.[1]

—*Carol Stepanchuk and Charles Wong,* Mooncakes and Hungry Ghosts

When tea is made with water,
drawn from the depths of the spirit,
of which the bottom is unfathomable,
then we have truly realized what is called
cha-no-yu [the tea ceremony].[2]

—*Toyotomi Hideyoshi*

As one of the its most ancient cultures, China has gifted the world with a vast array of gastronomic delights and food-related festivities, as well as the pleasures of tea. Yet underlying its immense culinary gifts are the even deeper meanings China has attributed to food: a harmonious bond between humankind and nature, a vehicle for social interaction, and an offering of reciprocity and communication between earthly human and heavenly spiritual beings. In celebrating the arrival of the new year, for example, the Chinese create carefully prepared meals and treats to welcome and win the favor of the hundreds of gods who are believed to visit their homes solely on this special night. As with this food ceremony, so filled with spiritual symbolism, the **Japanese Way of Tea** (Chanoyu) integrates the spiritual with the secular in one simple yet profound act—preparing and enjoying tea. With roots in Taoism, but originating with Zen Buddhist monks as a method of self-realization, the Japanese Way of Tea—often referred to in the West as the Japanese tea ceremony—developed in Japan in the fifteenth century as a way to enhance aesthetic exercises.[3] Today, China's New Year food festivities and Japan's Way of Tea have much in common. For both are centuries-old traditions with social harmony as the main ingredient, seasoned with spiritual significance.[4]

Kitchen Godliness

It is the "Little New Year" *(Xiaonian)* in homes throughout Hong Kong, one week before *Yuan Tan,* the festive New Year. A picture of the Kitchen God, or Lord of the Hearth *(Tsao-Chun),* has been resting the entire year on a shelf of each family's stove, which is believed to be the "soul" of the family, and arbiter of peace or strife.[5]

From his exalted position, the wooden Kitchen God has been observing the family members closely all year. But now it is time for the grandfather of the family to place the Kitchen God on an altar, ply the Kitchen God with sweet cakes and preserves, and prepare him for his annual ascent to the heavens. By "sweetening" him, the family hopes that when the Kitchen God ascends, he will report only good things about the people in the household to the revered Jade Emperor *(Yuhuangdi)* who waits in the heavens for the Kitchen God's report.

To send him off, the family takes the Kitchen God outside, then sets him on fire. At the same time, to ward off evil spirits, the family lights fireworks. As the smoke from the fire drifts upward toward heaven, they recite a prayer of hope:

> *Ascend to Heaven and speak of good things;*
> *Send blessings down to the world below....*[6]

For the next seven days—until the eve of the New Year—the shelf on the stove that houses the Kitchen God will remain empty. When New Year's Eve arrives, the grandfather will place a new image of the Kitchen God deity on the shelf. As with each prior year, it will remain on the shelf throughout the year, observing the family until it is his time to report their behavior to the Jade Emperor in the heavens during the next "Little New Year."

After the Kitchen God is in its place, the feast that is a midnight meal begins. And as it does, writes anthropologist Alain Y. Dessaint, so too does "the spiritual essence of the food satisf[y] the...spirits.[7]

A Midnight Meal for the Gods

Although the Kitchen God is pivotal to New Year festivities, the Chinese believe that hundreds of other gods will visit their homes on New Year's Eve to assess how the members of the family have behaved during the year. Based on pre-Confucian religious folklore, such beliefs date back thousands of years. According to China's ancient folk religion, food is a physical "bridge" between humans (earthly consciousness) and the gods (heavenly spirits). It is the vehicle whereby loving intentions and actions can be communicated to the gods and, in turn, reflected back to people via good fortune.

As we talked in a cafe, Suk Wah Bernstein, a writer living in Northern California, explained the intricacies of the New Year food offerings, derived from her memories about celebrating the New Year with her family during her childhood in Hong Kong.[8] "Chinese believe there is a god for each aspect of our lives. For instance, along with the Kitchen God, there is a god who guards the entrance to your door; a god who takes care of business; a righteousness god; a longevity god; one that gives us money; one for granting children; one for good fortune and prosperity....

"There's a god for just about everything. He or she comes to inspect you every now and then on his or her own schedule. However, on the eve of the Chinese New Year, all of them come. It's of paramount importance to welcome the hierarchy of gods and god-desses with the best you have. The preparation begins several days before. All the images are sparkling, the altars are washed and sparkling, and the grandmother makes sure that the best ingredients are set aside for preparing the special food for offering at 11:30 PM."

This midnight ritual is called *Kunzai* in Chinese. "The name of the meal carries a certain holiness to it," explains Bernstein. *Kun* means "offering with both hands and with great devotion and reverence. *Zai* is the Chinese character for vegetarian food.

"Earlier in the evening, the family gathers to have an elaborate meal. Soon afterward," continues Bernstein, "Grandma scrutinizes every corner of the house, especially the altars. Much as we think they are spotless, she unfailingly discovers tainted spots. Each member of the family is bathed and washed and wearing new clothes. Everyone is excited. After all, the gods, the inspectors, are coming."

At the same time, "the children and grandchildren have the opportunity to help with washing and chopping the vegetables for the *Zai*, but it is only Grandma—the matriarch of the family—who has the privilege of cooking them in accordance with tradition. When the vegetables are ready, she places the food on the main altar—because at 11:30 PM the gods will come around to inspect us. This is actually the first hour of the new year, and the food is a midnight offering to the gods who are coming around to check on the human world.

"This is the most important evening of the year," adds Bernstein, "because if you did anything bad during the year, this is your chance to receive the blessings of the gods and great fortune for the coming year. For instance, the spirit of the Righteousness God could visit this evening and correct any injustice in your life. You feel hope, ready to move forward. After all, this is the time when the gods are very easily pleased and they can't deny your wishes.

"In this spirit, the food is first presented at the main altar. Different families have different altars, some big, some small, some elaborate, some simple. There are different altars for different gods throughout the house. The type and number of altars depend on how worshipful the family members are toward the different gods."

Food Fit for the Gods

"Throughout China, all the food for the midnight meal is vegetarian food that has been dried or is fresh," continues Bernstein. "On one level, this is a festive family occasion, but its true essence is that you're revealing your devotion and trust in God; you are taking refuge in God. You do this by offering the best that you have to the gods. For the Chinese, what could be better than feeding the gods with their favorite food?

"The gods don't eat meat; this is why you prepare vegetarian food for them. They also require freshly made food, so the food is offered to them directly from the stove—while the life-force in the food is still full and strong.

"When I was a child, my eyes would focus on the *Zai*. There really was something delicious about that vegetarian dish she would make for that particular meal. My grandmother cooked it with much love and devotion, convinced that she was cooking for all the gods and goddesses that would protect us and bring fortune to her family and her children."

Midnight Offerings

The midnight vegetarian dish on which Bernstein would focus as her grandmother cooked, often included an array of vegetables that ranged from shiitake mushrooms and bean curd to Chinese broccoli and onions. Before sitting down to enjoy the meal, the most senior member of the family—usually the grandfather—would present food offerings to the gods at the altar and ask for protection, forgiveness, and blessings for any family member who had neglected to do what he or she should have during the year.

"He would do this by holding the food in both hands," says Bernstein, "with the left hand holding the right hand. And as he did this, my grandmother would pour 'God's wine'—special wine used in

China for worshipping the gods—into a little wine cup. My grandfather would take this wine cup, offer it to the gods, then sprinkle some on the ground in front of the entire altar.

"Then he would get on his knees and thank all the gods for coming to visit us. He would apologize for any wrongdoing during the year, ask them for compassion, and request that they look after us during the upcoming year. Along with the blessings is the hope that when the spirits descend to earth to inspect us at 11:30, they will catch us preparing great food for them, the best food. We hope that when they see the way we are honoring them with such good food, the gods will 'wipe out' whatever wrongdoings anyone did during the year."

In Bernstein's household, her grandmother "would fill up small offering bowls with *Zai*, then place them on a tray," she told me. "Then Grandma and Grandpa, together, would go to each altar in the house, place a bowl of food on each one, and offer some wine. The other family members would stand in silence as they did so. Meanwhile, the aroma of the *Zai* would permeate everywhere—along with the blessings of the gods and goddesses."

Spiritual Symbolism

Over the centuries, having a midnight meal with dear ones has become commonplace throughout China. As a matter of fact, Bernstein told me that there are restaurants that are open throughout the night to service people wishing to share a midnight meal. "Meeting in the middle of the night to dine is not a conscious connection to the new year," she says. "But I would say it's very much influenced by this tradition."

"The midnight meal is in my heart and soul," she adds, "because I grew up with it. If it's a good time for the gods to come around, it must be a good time for people, too." After all, "you're expressing your love for your friends—that they're family in your heart. Isn't this what spirituality is all about—to get connected with your heart and others?"

Of Leaves and Water

Agile Fingers
    pick a thousand buds.
Soon the scent of tea
    will fill the air.
Patience. My mind not yet quiet
    as it counts the Moments.
Ahh. The leaves are dancing
    so beautifully in the water![9]

—David Lee Hoffman,
proprietor, Silk Road Teas

Tea leaves in water. Legend tells us that tea as a beverage was created when a leaf from a nearby bush drifted into a cup of hot water. An obsolete Chinese emperor, who owned the cup, sipped, then savored the brew, and a new beverage was born.[10]

The symbolism of the Chinese New Year's midnight meal has entered the hearts of many Chinese people. But the role that *tea* has played throughout China since it became a valued beverage in the eighth century has even more significance. Over the centuries, throughout China, the enjoyment of drinking tea as well as its cultivation is similar to what the cultivation of grapes and wine is to the French—both an art and a passion.

Says David Lee Hoffman, proprietor of Silk Road Teas in Lagunitas, California, who travels to China twice yearly to select hundreds of hand-picked varietals of tea, "A good tea should be like fine wine. It should have a wide spectrum of activity when it hits your tongue. If you have a tea that has a personality to it, a pleasant personality, it's like enjoying a nice painting. Every time you drink it, you see different things.

"But there's more to tea than leaf and water. It's about savoring the moment as well as the tea. The beauty of tea is its simplicity. You put the tea leaves in water...and then the flavor of the tea is released into the hot water."

I spoke with Hoffman about his exotic, full-leaf, quality teas at his office. He is the first American to have ventured into remote areas of China to cultivate his own and others' tea gardens for export back to the United States. "Tea has a much greater significance in Asian cultures than it does in the States," he explained. "Asians greet and welcome people with tea. You quench your thirst with tea. You quiet your mind with tea. You stay awake with tea. You would never sit with anyone in Asia without a cup of tea in front of you."

Hearing the Silence, Seeing the Invisible

While enjoying and sharing tea is integral to Chinese culture, it is Japan's Way of Tea *(Chanoyu)*—designed to enrich both body and soul—that elevated tea to the realm of spiritual art in the fifteenth and sixteenth centuries. Writes Urasenke Grand Tea Master Sen Soshitsu XV: *"Chado,* the Way of Tea, is based on the simple act of boiling water, making tea, offering it to others, and drinking of it ourselves. Served with a respectful heart and received with gratitude, a bowl of tea satisfies both physical and spiritual thirst."[11]

Specifically, *chanoyu* refers to both the physical items (hot water, tea, tea bowls, etc.) and personal behavior connected to the formal imbibing of powdered green tea, while *chado* describes the spiritual path followed by practitioners of *chanoyu.*

Entering a Japanese teahouse *(chashitsu)* is comparable to enveloping oneself in perfect, harmonious, beautiful music. In the well-orchestrated, well-practiced simplicity within a Japanese tea house, visitors are invited to hear the subtle notes that play upon our finest feelings. In the teahouse, "we listen to the unspoken, we gaze upon the unseen," writes tea master Kakuzo Okakura in his classic *The Book of Tea.*[12] "The master calls forth notes we know not of. And in the process, we are participating in *teaism,* what Okakura describes as "a religion of aestheticism"[13] and the art of life.

Surrounded by the Japanese Way of Tea's timeless refinement, the pleasure we derive lies in the unfolding of subtle notes played throughout the ceremony that create an aesthetically simple but soul-satisfying experience. At any one time, we may hear the pouring of water, the clink of the lid on the iron kettle, or the whisking of the powdered green tea as it is turned into a light, frothy brew. The next moment may present the flat tone of the placement of the tea bowl onto the mat, the ongoing, varied cadences inherent in conversation, or the silence between the notes.

To experience the harmony of the Japanese Way of Tea firsthand, I visited the Nichibei Kai Culture Center, a three-story building in San Francisco's Japantown area. Representing ongoing friendship between the United States and Japan, the Center houses an authentic teahouse on the third floor. To enhance intimacy, the teahouse is small, and its natural materials preserve the beauty and simplicity of nature that is inherent in all teahouses.

When Mrs. Tsuruko Sekino, my host for the ceremony, learned I was interested in writing about the spiritual essence inherent in the Way of Tea, she invited her daughter Emiko Sekino to join us. Currently a graduate student at Thunderbird, the American Graduate School of International Management in Glendale, Arizona, Emiko has been learning the Way of Tea from her grandmother and mother since she was eight years old. Because of the hundreds of steps involved in the practice of tea—its preparation, distribution, and consumption—it is a lifetime endeavor.

"There is the outside world and then there is the world inside the tearoom," Emiko Sekino told me. "Inside the tearoom, we are interested in relationships, nonjudgmental socializing. The tearoom is designed to promote serenity and the idea of nature and people joining together."

Over the centuries, the Way of Tea has become more than a symbol of social interaction. It has also evolved into a master art, designed to enhance religio-aesthetic knowledge. This is evident in the common term *chado*, explained Emiko, which is often used to describe the Way of Tea. *Cha* means "tea"; the second syllable, *do*, has its roots in the Chinese philosophy/religion of the Tao.

Indeed, such a Zen approach to the practice of tea derives from the philosophy of *Taoism,* meaning "Way," the Absolute, or Nature. "The Tao is the passage rather than the path,"[14] writes Okakura. And within the Way is an appreciation of aesthetics, a philosophy that pertains to forms of beauty. Nowhere is this more evident than in the elements of the Way of Tea: the placement of flowers, scrolls with handmade calligraphy, the profound simplicity of the pottery, the architecture of the teahouse, and, of course, the tea powder itself.

But while Taoism provided the aesthetic ideals inherent in the Way of Tea, it was Zen, with its "conception of greatness in the smallest incidents of life,"[15] writes Okakura, that turned the Way of Tea into a practical pursuit. It was a southern Zen Buddhist sect, Okakura explains, that integrated many Taoist doctrines, originating the Way of Tea that is practiced today. These Zen monks, who gathered before the holy image of Bodhidharma to drink tea from a single bowl, infused the drinking of tea "with the profound formality of a holy sacrament."[16]

Evolved from the many art forms that were seen as a way to serenity, detachment, and peace of mind in fifteenth-century Japan, at its core, the Way of Tea is designed to allow the mystery, joy, and beauty within our hearts to spring forth. Some would describe it as a refuge from the "outside world," one that encourages an encounter with our Buddha nature. Consider this interpretation of the Way of Tea, written more than five hundred years ago by tea master Takuan:

The way of cha-no-yu ... *is to appreciate the spirit of a naturally harmonious blending of Heaven and Earth, to see the pervading presence of the five elements by one's fireside, where the mountains, rivers, rocks, and trees are found as they are in nature, to draw the refreshing water from the well of Nature, to taste with one's own mouth the flavor supplied by nature.*[17]

Elements of Tea

When most of us consider the elements that make up a Japanese tea gathering, we tend to conjure up images of tea bowls, the kettle, and the tea itself. But for practitioners of the Way of Tea, the concept of *elements* is much broader. Indeed, these physical elements are not the only "notes" that are necessary to participate in the "symphony." The artistry that goes into the creation of the various elements also contributes to the harmony of the experience.

Christy A. Bartlett's interest in the various elements of the Way of Tea began when she was an American student studying art in Japan.[18] Today, she is the founding director of the San Francisco branch of the Urasenke Foundation, and a disciple of Sen Soshitsu XV, head of the Foundation and the fifteenth-generation descendant of venerated tea master Rikyu (1522–1591). While preserving the traditions begun by his ancestors, Sen Soshitsu XV has opened the study of the Way of Tea to non-Japanese people at his centers worldwide.

Says Bartlett, "The study of tea is vast. People who study the subject usually select an area that appeals to them most. While there is a broad knowledge that one must have, each person may specialize in a particular area." For some, this may mean approaching the practice of tea as a study of Zen—either as a student or a teacher. Others may specialize in ceramics, landscape design, or studying the history as an art historical project. "Or even the history of one particular potter," continues Bartlett. "Or tea gardens, tea architecture, or literature about tea."

Adds Scott McDougall, a student of the Way of Tea at the Urasenke Foundation, "People who study tea may benefit from both the physical practice and the intellectual stimulation of various specialties." This is so "because tea is an art form one may practice for a lifetime without exhausting its possibilities."

As significant as the "seeable" elements are, four basic "unseeable" principles developed by Rikyu contribute equally to the aesthetics of the tea experience. They include: *wa*, harmony among people, nature, and the way in which people use the tea utensils; *kei*, authentic respect and appreciation for others; *sei*, both worldly and spiritual purity; and *jaku*, serenity that comes with the understanding of *wa*, *kei*, and *sei*.[19]

What follows are some of the "physical" elements integral to tea ceremonies which, along with the four basic principles, are integral to promoting a sense of serenity, strengthening the bonds of friendship, and satisfying the senses. By filling the senses with beauty, the elements also offer an opportunity for each visitor to "cleanse the... senses of any impurities," writes Eelco Hesse in *Tea: The Eyelids of Bodhidharma*.[20]

Landscape garden. Walking on the path through the garden that leads to the tea room is the beginning of the ceremony. It is the first stage of disconnecting from the outside world.

The entrance. The entrance that leads into the tea room is only three feet high. Therefore, entering the tea room calls for bowing down— a symbol of humility.

Placement of flowers. Representing the sense of smell, the flower also represents the season in which the ceremony is taking place. The flower is placed *(ireru)* rather than arranged *(ikeru)* in a special flower vase *(hana-ire)*, reflecting the type of tea ceremony that is occurring.

Hanging scroll. Hanging above the floral arrangement in the alcove (the *tokonoma*, the heart of the tearoom) is a scroll that contains Japanese calligraphy, usually painted in ink. The words on the scroll reflect the theme of the particular tea ceremony.

Utensils. Arranged harmoniously, an array of varied utensils are used throughout the ceremony. The teaspoon, frequently made of bamboo or lacquer, is used to scoop the powdered green tea from the canister into the tea bowl.

Kettle. To fill the sense of hearing, both the boiling and pouring of the water create sound during the ceremony. The kettle is typically made of iron, occasionally of bronze. The lid of the kettle has a special stand *(futaoki)* on which it rests.

Tea bowl. The tea bowl plays a major role throughout the Way of Tea. During the winter, thick bowls are used to keep tea warm; in warmer months, shallower bowls serve to cool the tea.

Green tea. Zen monks brought powdered green tea to Japan centuries ago. When whisked together with hot water, the green powder becomes thick and foamy. To enhance the look of the tea, it is often served in black bowls.

Tea whisk. Used to whip the powdered tea and water into a frothy mixture, the tea whisk (*cha-sen*) is intricately carved of bamboo.

Cultivating Tea Mind

As much as it is an actual ceremony filled with elements, the Way of Tea is also a consciousness, a "mentality of elegance," an ability to appreciate the beauty of the elements—from the singing of the water as it is poured into the bowl to the natural sounds of the human voice and the ebb and flow of conversation as ideas, reactions, and emotions are expressed. It is truly an experiential adventure that unfolds along with the passing moments.

So integral are the aesthetics of the Way of Tea in Japanese culture, the concept has even infiltrated the language. For instance, the word *chajin* describes a person who has internalized the spiritual ideals of the Way of Tea—both while preparing tea and in everyday existence. As a contrast, a person with an inability to appreciate such aesthetics is sometimes described as a person "without tea"; the converse also applies: those with an excessive amount of free-flowing emotions may be described as having "too much tea."[21]

Consider the message on the hanging scroll that is designed to enhance conversation, aesthetic appreciation of the tea experience, and "tea mind." When I visited Bartlett and McDougall at the Urasenke Foundation's teahouse, Bartlett was kind enough to translate the Japanese calligraphy: "Unself-consciousness leads back to the greater path." In a typical tea ceremony, "one would never pose a point-blank question such as, 'What is the meaning of this scroll?'" she explained. Rather, "one is appreciative in an open way that invites explications, and one savors the slow unfolding of the answer. The scrolls, however, always present a topic that people comment upon."

Ultimately, the entire experience — "the making of tea, the drinking of tea, and the taste of tea — are a means toward an intellectual and artistic experience. This reflects the Japanese culture in many ways. It is at once extremely down-to-earth, and yet what is down-to-earth and everyday is not denied in importance or depth of meaning."

Brewing Spiritual Sustenance

Philosopher Huston Smith tells us that "trying to understand the human story without religion would be like trying to explain smoke without fire."[22] In the same light, participating in a tea ritual or the Way of Tea without resonating with the underlying meaning is like reading a beautiful poem for its mere words.

Ultimately, the Way of Tea is constructed of principles that transcend any particular culture, embodying the spiritual marriage of art with nature, of "everydayness" with sacred pursuits. The physical and spiritual elements of the tea ceremony, and the way in which they "play" together to satisfy the senses, create an introspective sensibility that is the essence of the Zen philosophy.

Journeying to this sacred center may last during the moments in which we partake of tea — or we may carry it within our being for a day, week, month, or lifetime. For tea is more than a sublime beverage. When savored with a "tea mind," it becomes a true alchemical brew from which flows a cornucopia of spiritual sustenance.

Celebrating Midnight Meals,
Cultivating Tea Consciousness

In the spirit of the Chinese New Year, "satisfy the spirits" in your own life by creating your own spiritually imbued midnight meal. You may do this on New Year's Eve or choose to celebrate what Bernstein has called "the magic of the night,"[23] any time the mood strikes. The intention: to create a celebratory midnight meal that regards the first hour of the day—the newness of the day, month, or year—and to celebrate this special "transition" time with loved ones.

"Invite friends to come over to your home for a midnight supper," Bernstein suggests. "You can do this any night. Do it spontaneously. You don't want to put too much planning into it." The purpose is to "have a long midnight chat, to open up your heart with each other," says Bernstein. "There's a quality in the night that brings up something that has been buried during the day. And there's also some power in the night itself...that takes you over the threshold of the constraints of the mundane world."

To experience such "otherworldliness," Bernstein offers the following suggestions for manifesting your own magical midnight meal and communicating with beneficent gods.

Managing the meal

Be informal. When you invite someone to a midnight supper in your home, avoid a dress code in order to minimize and break through formalities. Given the time and occasion, participating in "the magic of the night" is an invitation to open up.

Cook lightly. Because of the time of day, make a dish that is light and easily digested. Begin cooking when your friends arrive.

Keep it simple. Use whatever food is available in your kitchen. For instance, if you find some pasta in your pantry and some vegetables in your refrigerator, consider making a pasta dish with a vegetable-based sauce. Serving the food directly from the stove—while it's still warm—communicates comfort and enhances a sense of connectedness.

Garnering the gods

Make a welcoming, soothing atmosphere. Consider dimming the lights and lighting some candles instead of using overhead lighting.

Create a theme. To communicate with the gods during the midnight meal, consider developing a theme for the night. Perhaps a friend just had a promotion at work, has a personal problem, or is simply bored. Invite him or her over to celebrate or discuss the situation.

Select a spirit. Based on the meal's theme, define the gods or goddesses with whom you wish to communicate.

Say affirmations. During the meal, say some prayers or affirmations about your situation.

Preparing Mind and Leaves

Some would say that the delicacy of the tea ritual no longer fits into the often frenzied pace of the Western world. But it *is* possible to slow down life and create the unhurried, authentic experience of a tea ritual by becoming a *chajin* (one of "tea mind"), if only for a few moments. It calls for a willingness to participate in the spiritual path inherent in the practice of the Way of Tea, as well as cultivating a particular consciousness and basic tea-making skills.

In Japan, tea masters are likely to use powdered tea, while those in China use tea leaves that are brewed. Although becoming a tea master entails years of practice and study—often a lifetime—Chinese tea proprietor David Hoffman offers this perspective for simulating the Oriental tea experience without extensive training: "A tea master is someone who can prepare the perfect cup of tea with complete awareness." The five qualities of steeped tea [taste, aroma, the appearance of the leaf before and after steeping, and water] are a small part of the experience compared to the entire world you create among yourself, your guests, and the tea. This world is one of tranquility, respect, and honor."

To create this world in your own home, here are some of Hoffman's suggestions for preparing both mind and tea:

Preparing "mind"

Create an environment that is clean, unpretentious, simple, fresh, and tranquil. By creating a clean, serene environment and serving your best tea in your best ware, you are offering both yourself and your guests the best that you can.

Keep motion to a minimum while preparing the tea. Refrain from making movements that have nothing to do with the preparation and serving of the tea.

Prepare the tea while your guests are present. Making the tea mindfully is an expression of the appreciation of the process. To show respect, use your finest tea for guests, with your finest utensils and wares.

Empty your mind of idle chatter. Engage in pleasant conversation, without rambling on and on or jumping from one topic to another.

Focus on the preparation, presentation, and enjoyment of the tea. In this way, you're quieting the mind.

Preparing tea

Tea pot. Quality teapots are made of porous clay; they are not glazed. (The best teapots in the world are from Yixing, China, notes Hoffman.) Because they absorb the flavor of the tea, over time, the teapot will develop its own character. Preheat the teapot with hot water.

Water. Steel kettles are for heating water. The amount of water you use varies, as do the varietals of tea. Let your own palate be your guide.

Tea leaf. Although there are more than two hundred varietals of what Hoffman calls "pure tea," the major categories include green tea (the leaf is rolled); black tea (the leaves oxidize for twelve to fourteen hours); oolong tea (the leaves are partially oxidized); and white tea (the leaves are the least processed; they are air-dried or steamed). During the Way of Tea, the Japanese most often use powdered green tea.

When brewing the tea leaves, first consider the size of the teapot. Hoffman recommends about six grams (⅕ oz.) of tea for a twelve-ounce teapot. "You can't go by volume," he says, "because some tea is very light; other tea is heavy." Experiment until you find the proportion of tea to water that is most pleasing for you.

Temperature. Boiling water destroys most green and white teas. Hoffman suggests the following temperatures for optimal flavor: white or green (70°–75° C); oolongs (80°–90° C); black (near boiling).

Brewing. To allow the flavor to develop fully, brew tea loosely; avoid tea balls or infusers. Your own personal flavor preference will determine the amount of time in which the tea should brew. Consider taste rather than color.

Finally, Hoffman suggests savoring "the beautiful colors and shapes of the leaves while brewing, because appearance is very much a part of the experience."

nine

Native American: The Vision Quest Fast

The process by which inner strength grows at the expense of physical strength during a period of... fasting... and searching is as familiar to the... Hindu, Buddhist, Christian, Islamic, or Jewish scripture as it is to the American Indian on his vision quest.[1]

—*Mircea Eliade*

It is through the vision quest, participated in with physical sacrifice and the utmost humility, that the individual opens himself... to contact with the spiritual essences. Often the sacred experience comes in the mysterious appearance of an animal or a winged being... A special message is often communicated to the seeker, and this will serve as a guide and reminder throughout the person's life.[2]

—*Joseph Epes Brown*,
Animals of the Soul

Virtually every religion worldwide turns to fasting as an outward expression of a spiritual pursuit that is believed to purge both body and soul of sin, guilt, and defilement—and to encourage a sense of purity. Continuing the tradition of Moses, who fasted for forty days on Sinai in service to God, devout Jews observe **Yom Kippur** by abstaining from food on the Day of Atonement; as Jesus did for forty days before embarking on his ministry, modern-day Christians fast by observing **Lent**, a time of penitence; and Muslims fast during

Ramadan, a month-long fast that is designed to enhance spiritual growth and discipline, and express devotion to the divine.

But fasting is not only an act of penitence. Native American hunting tribes observe a *vision quest fast* as preparation for communion with the spiritual, a way to receive knowledge and guidance. As with other fasting traditions, the vision quest is a centuries-old ecstatic discipline, a spiritual journey that opens the sojourner to greater receptivity to visions and dreams, and communion with divine "knowing."

Guardian Spirits and Vision Quests

For thousands of years, people from Eastern and Western cultures have borne testimony to the link between fasting and transcendence, visionary truths, and life renewal. Fasting—the custom of abstaining from nourishment—is virtually a universal phenomenon practiced by those on a spiritual quest who seek guidance, purification, or supplication through contact with the divine. For instance, ancient Greco-Roman schools of philosophy favored fasting as a means to commune and connect with the spiritual; Taoism teaches the concept of *hsin-chai,* fasting from the heart (rather than the body), to arrive at the Tao; and followers of Confucianism fasted to prepare for worship of ancestral spirits.[3]

But while many religious adherents fast to atone for sins, members of Native American hunting tribes view abstaining from food as a core aspect of the vision quest—an opportunity to receive guidance from the Great Spirit, the Creator. When braves set out for a forest or wilderness to pursue a ritual fast in solitude, they are seeking a transformative vision, insights into the direction various aspects of their lives should take. Ideally, the message will appear as a personal vision to seekers via a *guardian spirit,* often in the guise of a bird or animal who brings blessings, insights, and "knowledge to the soul" of its human ally. Such is the potential power of the Native American spiritual fast. For as the sensual stimulation of food diminishes, our awareness turns toward the life force that created food, us...and the message from our "guardian spirits."

Fasting with the Eagle

What follows is the experience of the vision quest of Native American Katie Martin, mother of six and grandmother of thirteen. Katie's mother is part Sioux and part Mohawk, her father Sioux and Ojibwa. It was only recently that Katie learned of her mother's Sioux heritage when Katie's sister found their maternal grandmother's handwritten autobiography in the pocket of an old apron. It was then that they discovered that their grandmother had been adopted as a child by the Sioux tribe of Six Nations, Canada.

Katie's husband, David, is a spiritual leader *(Shaman)* who has dedicated his life to healing others. When they married more than thirty years ago, Katie chose to go on a vision quest "to find out what it meant to be a part of my husband's life," she told me during a phone conversation. "I wanted to do more than just stand by him. I wanted to find out how to be involved...to be a part of what he was doing." With the help the guardian spirit sent to her by what she calls "Creator," she received a visionary truth and an answer to her quest.

"With Creator's help, I decided to fast to find out if I was going to dedicate my whole life to my husband's work as a spiritual healer. To do this, I wanted to cleanse my mind, to cleanse my body, to purify my whole being. To show Creator that I was serious about being more than David's wife, I gave up food for four days so that I would be in a spiritual and humble frame of mind when I talked to Creator. By fasting and going into the woods away from everybody, we can get back to Mother Nature. This is how it was a long time ago...when you could focus and be with Creator and all living things and animals.

"I started the fast at midnight, although I didn't go into the woods until the next morning, which is when the person who would be watching over me would be free. The day before he came over, I was fortunate to have an Elder lady guide me through the fast. She was the one who told me to start at midnight, and to be sure that I got my colors [bags filled with sacred tobacco], so that I could set them out in the four directions for Creator to see. The four colors are white, yellow, red, and either black or blue. They represent the four colors of the Nation of People: red people, black people, yellow people, and white people.

"Tobacco is sacred to us. We pray with it and use it for prayers. As with the bread and wine in the Eucharist for Christians, we use tobacco when we talk to Creator. I put the tobacco in the pouches in the four colors as an offering to Creator, then hung them up by a nearby tree. Sometimes you have an offering tree, and you put them up there. You're offering the tobacco and colors up to Creator to let Him know how serious you are about what you're doing.

"My friend came to get me at my house in the morning before he went to work, then he took me into the woods and 'smudged me down.' Before we do anything that we consider sacred, special, or good—or if we're asking for guidance—we'll burn a smudge. A smudge is a 'stick' or balls of sacred herbs—often sage—that we use to pray. As far back as I can remember, when I was a little child, my grandmother and the Elders always told us that sage was sent by Creator to the Indian people to use to pray with.

"There are lots of different kinds of sage that grow wild in the wilderness. We pick it and dry it, then wrap it or shred it right off the stem. From this we make a stick from strands of sage, then we wrap them together with yarn; other times, we'll make them into a ball, then burn the balls of sage. We light the sage sticks or balls to create smoke and talk to Creator. The smoke symbolizes that there is life in that smoke—that Creator made it. I put the smoke all over my body. You start from the top of your head, all the way down your body. Basically, you're purifying your body with the smoke. To make a smudge means that you're asking for some time to talk with Creator. It's very sacred to us. When I'm praying and I've got a smudge going, my kids and grandkids know to leave me alone because that's my time with God.

"After my friend came to get me and bring me into the woods, he smudged me down. He did this by lighting sage and putting the smoke all over my body...to purify my body and mind. I received the smudging as a blessing and was thankful for that. Because it's always an honor when someone does this to you. I appreciated that he was getting me ready to fast and be out there with Creator.

"I was by myself the whole time except for the one time when my friend came by to bring me water and make sure I was safe. I was alone in the forest in a sweat lodge in a wooded area outside of Minneapolis. Although the sweat lodge is used to purify and cleanse your body and spirit with the heat, I used it for shelter. I didn't eat any food at all. I only drank water, and I only drank it in the morning.

"I sat and prayed and talked with Creator, asking him to help me understand what my job was with David. What was my life with him and how did I fit in? What was it He wanted me to do? I did this because my husband had been learning to be a spiritual leader. He was given the ability, the authority, blessings, and permission to do this from the Elder who taught him to do different things.

"While David was learning, I had been learning things on my own, too. By fasting and asking Creator for guidance, I wanted to learn if I was meant to be involved in what David was doing—helping and healing others.

"While I prayed, I focused on nature—the trees, earth, animals, birds. I slept and rested and drank water, but I only drank water once a day—first thing in the morning. And I sang songs that we [Native Americans] sing in prayer meetings. There are some songs I wasn't quite sure of, so I asked Creator to help me out with those.

"Creator gave me the knowledge I asked for. He showed me what I wanted to know by sending me the eagle, which is the spirit." *At this point in our conversation, Katie was silent for a moment for she was moved to tears of joy and appreciation as she recalled the presence of this guardian spirit—and the spiritual gift that the Creator had sent to her.*

"We believe that Creator has blessed us with animals in our life to guide us, show us, support us, protect us, and watch over us. The eagle especially helps the people spiritually. While I was fasting, the eagle came over and just sat there in a nearby tree, watching me during that time. Because of its presence, I felt I was doing the right thing. It stayed with me the whole time, but when I woke up on the fourth day, the eagle was gone. This is how I knew I was finished with my fast. I was feeling connected with everyday life again . . . not feeling spiritual anymore.

"The night before the eagle left, as I was sleeping I had a dream. My husband came to me in my dream and told me to come home, that the fast is over. I believe that Creator used him to tell me it was time to come home. But first I had to wait for my friend who would come for me in the afternoon after work.

"What I learned was that David and I could fit together like a puzzle, and that we could work together this way. There were things He was showing David and things He was showing me. And there are things that David's good at, and things that I'm good at. Together, we could make the puzzle whole. This meant He wanted me to be here for the people, to help my husband in doctoring by supporting him morally and spiritually . . . and to be a part of that spiritual help.

"I was more positive after I realized this. I was strong—spiritually, physically, and in every way that you can think of. I was able to connect with Creator at all times, not just from two to four o'clock; I mean *all* the time. I now live with an awareness that Creator is my whole life. My kids know that it's me and Creator; then me and my husband; then me and the children and my grandkids. Creator is my whole life and my husband knows this, because it's his whole life. He's fasted too. Fasting is how he got to where he is today.

"Fasting helped us to understand that the purpose of our life is to be one with Creator at all times. We are dedicated to Him—not just talking about it, but doing it."[4]

Fasting with the Goat

Every three years since 1989, my husband, Larry Scherwitz, has embarked on a vision quest. For him, it takes the form of an intensive, spiritual fast in the Weminuche (pronounced "whim-in-nooch"), a four million acre wilderness area in southwestern Colorado that was the hunting grounds for the Ute Indians hundreds of years ago.

During his fasting retreat in September 1995, Larry spent an extraordinary thirty-six hours with a feisty white mountain goat, which he believes was "a guardian spirit sent to give me strength and steadfastness during the fast and quest." Indeed, in the Hindu tradition, the goat symbolizes the higher self.[5] Keeping notes of the experience by journaling in his tent, Larry created what he has come to call his "goat notes." What follows are excerpts from these notes—and a glimpse into the spiritual insights Larry derived during an auspicious, memorable visit from his "guardian messenger."

Day 1

"It is 3:30 in the morning, and I am writing by candlelight, recalling that I had been awakened from yesterday afternoon's nap by a stomping sound outside of my tent. When I raised my head, cobralike, to peer outside, looking directly at me was a large, beautiful all-white mountain goat, standing confidently not more than twelve feet from the tent entrance. He was so clean and white, so regal in his stance, so perfectly groomed and formed—in the prime of his life—and unafraid of me. Most powerful of all was his gaze, which was transfixed on me.

"Fascinated, I had carefully unzipped the tent, crept out, and slowly walked toward him. At a closer distance, I saw that all four of his hooves were positioned in the center of the prayer circle of rocks that I had made during the 1989 vision quest, six years before. What was the significance of his standing in this prayer circle? Was he a spiritual figure, sent in the form of an animal? I felt so. I would call him 'Freddy.'

"As he grazed in different locations around the campsite, I continued to position myself nearby—but at a respectful distance. His mostly black, powerful horns swooped backward, ending in a sharp point at the tips that could serve as a real weapon should he lower his head and use his strong legs and neck. Freddy stood about four feet high on his front legs; about three-and-a-half feet at his hind legs. I guessed that he weighed about 175 pounds. As I watched, I learned what he liked to eat: white paintbrush, blooming fireweed, and a nondescript low-lying plant with oval green leaves. For variety he pulled off the leaves of the salt willow, a hardy bush that grows above tree-line tundra.

"As I began to feel the coolness of the late afternoon and my own fatigue from fasting, I said a silent, heartfelt farewell to Freddy, then walked back to my tent. After ten minutes of relaxing in the warmth of the tent, I heard the sound of Freddy's hooves and knew he was just outside. Later, when I left the tent to get some water at the nearby lake, I noticed that Freddy positioned himself within sight of me. He remained still, silhouetted at sunset against the pink and blue colors in the sky. I was overcome by this beautiful sight, aware that the Great Spirit seemed to have answered my prayer of a few days earlier by bringing me into contact with a guardian spirit—in the form of an animal—during this quest.

"That evening, Freddy continued to watch me as I cleaned up and prepared for sleep. Throughout the night, he remained close to the tent site, mostly grazing; sometimes he was so close, I could hear him breathing. When I peered outside, I saw that even though the moon had set, Freddy's white coat remained brilliant in the natural starlight in the high altitude of the wilderness.

Day 2

"When I awakened at 6:30 the next morning, I looked outside the tent and found Freddy gazing directly at me as he again stood in my meditation spot. My impression: that he was in my 'spirit place.' When I asked the Creator why Freddy was here with me, I received the answer that he had been sent to bring energy and steadfastness to me during my spiritual quest. It was working, for I seemed to draw strength from Freddy's strength, and when I felt weak from the fast, I derived energy from him too.

"After realizing this, I approached Freddy. But this time, instead of continuing to gaze at me, he raised his head high, made a couple of sharp, loud exhalations, whined, backed up about fifteen feet, and then charged toward me—only to stop within five feet to rear up on his hind legs and make bucking motions by jutting his neck, head, and horns. For a split second I was alarmed, but then I projected loving energy as protection. After he stopped, I told him silently that I would play with him. He appeared to understand, for he began to prepare for the second round.

"In response, I backed up, snorted emphatically in sync with him, charged as he charged, raised myself up as he stood up on his back legs, and moved my head as if to butt my imaginary horns against his very real horns. We repeated this ritual two more times, stopping only because he decided not to play anymore. Instead, he chose to return to grazing. I pondered in deep awe about what had just happened between Freddy and me. Was it a challenge or play? Or was it a shared brotherhood?

"Suddenly it began to hail, and the pea-size hail stones pelted the ground softly. I didn't move, though. Instead, I chose to sit in place, feeling the depth of the new level of communication between Freddy and me. Perhaps the changing atmosphere brought by the approaching storm cloud and the cooler weather, had influenced him—as it did me.

"As the gentle hail turned to harsher rain and thunder, I took cover in my tent. I wasn't concerned about lightning on the exposed ridge where my tent was located because I thought that early fall thunderstorms would be gentler than the often violent summer ones. Then suddenly a brilliant flash of lightning and a simultaneous clap of thunder struck to the right of my tent in the direction of where Freddy was standing. As I listened to vestiges of the rumble, I waited with bated breath for another strike of lightning.

"Was there a message in the thunder and lightning bolt?

Northern Native Americans believe lightning and thunder represent the universal spirit, while *shamans* think the flash of lightning signifies a bridge between the spiritual and secular worlds.[6] I reflected on the last few days of fasting, solitude, and my goat companion; now nature had sent me a 'charged' message. I believe that fasting had opened my senses, leaving me in an altered state that filled me with respect, gratitude, and awe for both nature and Freddy, my spiritual guardian.

"When the rain stopped, I unzipped the tent and peered out: a wet Freddy was nearby—again gazing right at me.

Day 3

"I awoke the next morning to find Freddy standing in my meditation spot again. Later, though, I began to feel even weaker than yesterday, so much so that I could not sit upright to meditate, much less do yoga. Why was I so weak? Perhaps because after having spent three days doing strenuous, uphill hiking before fasting, I simply no longer had enough energy to make red blood cells and to adjust to the altitude; I had also been continually burning energy to keep warm. Concerned, I lay down, knowing I wouldn't have the energy to backpack the necessary nine miles out of the area, back to civilization, if I didn't recover strength. After all, it was a three thousand foot drop and a one thousand five hundred foot climb to the nearest road.

"The solution was obvious: I would break the fast, not only to recharge, but because the weakness was keeping me from doing my spiritual practices of yoga, meditation, and prayer. To begin, I prepared a cup of miso broth, then a cup of tea, then some potatoes. While I prepared the food, Freddy became skittish: he turned his face to the north and appeared to listen to something and to smell something. I followed his gaze, but neither heard, saw, or smelled anything.

"Then, just as I started to eat, Freddy jumped as if startled and descended down the nearby ledge. After eating, when I had gained enough strength, I searched for him by scouting the area for a half-mile radius all around. I even climbed to the highest point in the area, where I could see for a mile over the landscape in every direction. Surely, with his white coat, I could easily spot him. But Freddy was not to be seen; he had disappeared. I began to miss his presence.

"In retrospect, the fast and vision quest were spiritually affirming. The biggest lesson: that God answers prayers and responds to sacrificial efforts to form a deeper connection by providing the help that is needed. I also learned that all the activity we engage in has a deeper purpose than just the activity itself. For through our intentions and actions, we evolve into our way of being in the world. Another lesson: Sitting silently allows one to transcend layers of mental activity and thinking, and in their place, connect with intangible dreams and deep yearnings that emanate from the soul.

"The quest allowed me to experience how to just be in the world, rather than continually do things; but more important, it provided a spiritual path for getting there. Being with Freddy taught me this. He had his own way of simply being, and through observing his "being-ness," he pointed the way for me to realize my own way of being. In my mind's eye and in my heart, I know that this is the vision that fasting during the quest provided."

Gazing Between the Bites

While Larry fasted in the company of Freddy the goat, he noted that Freddy would graze for food by pulling off pieces of grass and flowers, then he would raise his head and gaze while chewing. In between bites, he would continue to chew while taking in the environment.

In such a way, fasting is an opportunity to experience a long, internal, insightful "gaze" in between our meals—whether the gaze occurs between daily meals or during a four-day fast. For in those moments when we are abstaining from nourishment—those moments that are devoid of food preparation, cooking, and cleaning up—we have the opportunity to gaze, as Freddy does, at both our external and inward "spiritual environment."

When we refrain from eating when surrounded by nature, the

mind turns to nature and our inner essence to replace the sensuality and stimulation normally provided by food. As "internal gazing" replaces unconscious "grazing," the creation that is our body/mind turns to contemplation and being in the moment. Instead of food, the scent of the air, the change in the weather—perhaps the guardian animal that has been sent to watch over us during the fast—become our nourishment. And in the process, we receive the true meaning inherent in fasting and the Native American vision quest: the timeless, all-embracing human experience of transcendence, a connection to nature, our self, and the silent sound that is the mystery of life itself.

Fundamentals of Fasting

People choose to abstain from food for a variety of reasons: as a rite of spiritual purification, penitence and purification, communion with God, or to enhance healing. For fasting to be a catalyst for spiritual transformation—rather than an experience of discomfort or anxiety—it's a good idea develop a personal plan. Here are some strategies:

Prepare for the fast. Deciding that you want to fast is the first step toward achieving it. Psychological and physical preparation is part of the process and ritual of fasting. Once you've prepared yourself psychologically to dedicate and allot a certain amount of time to the fast, you'll have a clearer understanding of the best setting and type of fast that's right for you.

Eliminate problem-causing food. To benefit from the time you spend fasting, eliminate "discomfort-causing" foods and liquids from your diet several days before you begin to fast. Some examples: coffee, tea, caffeine-containing colas, chocolate, excessive sweets, etc. Eliminating these drinks and foods from your diet may cause headaches, lethargy, and other uncomfortable symptoms for several days.

Clarify the type of fast. Do you intend to take a moderate approach to fasting, and refrain from eating during certain hours of the day (as is done during the Islamic Ramadan)? Or would you prefer to follow a juice fast that consists of various types of fruit and vegetable juice? The purest form of fasting, consisting of drinking only water, is a criteria of the vision quest fast. The type of fast you select depends on prior fasting experience, your health, and the intention of your fast. Because it provides calories and vitamins and minerals, the juice fast is often easier for novices.

Identify your intention. Why are you fasting? To commune with nature? Find a solution to a problem? Rest and heal? Develop a clearer perspective on what your path in life ought to be? To feel closer to God or solve a personal problem? Once you clarify your intention, it'll be easier for you to determine the duration of the fast, and the most appropriate environment in which to conduct it.

Choose a setting. The environment in which you fast should help you to achieve your goals. If possible, choose a setting that is conducive to opening you to sensory insights and new perspectives about your life. Whether fasting in nature or your home, choose a setting that is safe and familiar, so that you are free to experience spiritual insights.

Expect stages. When you first begin to fast, your body is still obtaining energy from recently eaten food. Depending on when you last ate, and how much, it will take time for your body physiology to slow down. At first, you may experience headaches, weakness, food cravings, or a sense of deprivation—especially if you typically drink caffeinated beverages such as coffee or colas. By the second day, these sensations are likely to diminish or stop, and be replaced with feelings of well-being and more physical strength.

Consider activities. Along with deciding to set aside time to fast and "detox," preparation also means planning the activities that will take place during your fast. Some examples of appropriate activities are meditating, creating a prayer circle, reading an inspirational book, or simply resting and staring at the sky. Another option is to make a prayer circle of rocks, each of which represents loved ones in your life. Then sit within the circle and focus on various stones as you say prayers for various people. The key concept is planning to be less active and relaxed, so that you are more open to signals you may receive from nature.

Keep a journal. Consider keeping a diary of your experiences throughout the day. Reflect upon, process, and record any insights or experiences you may have had. Journaling is one way of focusing and processing the underlying meaning of your fast. By staying alone and remaining aware of your thoughts and feelings, you are more likely to experience both the boredom and the ecstasy of the various stages of the fast.

Enhance spiritual awareness. Without the sensory stimulation of food, your thoughts, feelings, and soul are more likely to turn to, and open up to, spiritual subtleties. Without the satiety of food, your senses become keener, visual acuity sharpens, and aromas are more acute. As the body weakens, the soul seems to strengthen, making you more open to an experiential adventure—one that helps you to experience the unity of all life.

Break the fast. Fasting can provide an opportunity to give you a new perspective on what and how you usually eat. Before breaking the fast, consider any changes in your relationship to food. When you begin to eat again, choose small portions of easily digestible food, such as broth or soup. The longer you've fasted, the more time you'll need to take to build up to your usual diet.

ten

Hinduism:
The Wedding Feast

Men have always feasted, in huts and palaces and
temples, in an instinctive gesture of gratitude to
their gods.[1]

—M. F. K. Fisher

Traditional Hindus see the world as a hierarchy of
interpenetrating substances, and food ingested in the
body is a potent medium for transmitting psychic
substance between individuals.[2]

—Mircea Eliade

Perhaps more than at any other event, it is the food shared at
wedding feasts—by both the bridal couple and guests—that is lush
with sacred symbolism and celebratory sentiment. For instance,
food, considered hallow by the early Israelites, continues to be abundant at Jewish weddings as acknowledgment of God's hand in both
the union of the couple and the creation of the food itself. Indeed,
for most religions and cultures, food served at the wedding feast
emphasizes symbolism rather than spectacle: For a typical Polish
wedding feast, the Catholic church blesses the **kolacze,** a flat, plaited
loaf of bread that symbolizes all bread—the staff of life;[3] and
because the wedding feast represents the couple's future married
life, an abundance of good, solid, traditional food is often served at
Polish weddings.[4] What follows is an invitation to attend a **Hindu
wedding feast,** and witness the Hindu concept of **samskara,** a rite

that both consecrates and purifies the couple through the oblation of food with fire. Let us join the bride and groom as they exchange marriage vows—as food and fire interpenetrate to transmit blessings to the bride and groom, and set the stage for the fabulous, blessing-filled feast that follows.

Spiritually Flavored Food Offerings

The spiritual significance of the wedding feast in Hindu tradition is rooted in the *Vedas,* India's earliest religious literature that predates the *Bhagavad Gita.* The essence of the Vedic sacramental system can be expressed by the Latin phrase, *do ut des:* "I give that you may give," and the Sanskrit word *bhakti,* which signifies devotion to God and means to eat, partake of, and to love.[5] Ancient devotees were also asked to make offerings of food, drink, and spiritual veneration to the gods in exchange for health and prosperity.

Today, thousands of years after the *Vedas,* the tradition continues. Hindus who marry offer food both to the god of fire and to those who attend the wedding so that all may receive blessings. In this way, the food that is transformed by the fire-altar's open flame into rising smoke that feeds the gods also nourishes an internal spiritual fire, while the banquet itself becomes an offering that encourages blessings for both the couple and their families and friends. By examining the wedding feast, we can learn much about the food that feeds both body and soul.

Partaking in communal eating at wedding feasts is to share a sense of well-being and joy and exhilaration with the bride and groom. It is a meal of particular importance, for not only do friends and family share food, they do so as a temporary social group that has been created to grace and honor the newly married couple. Eating together. Sensing together. Consuming together. Communal sharing of food takes us out of ourselves and connects us to others. And as with the food-related wisdom traditions discussed in this book, we realize we are a part of the unifying life force in food and of those with whom we share food. Such is the connection and the sense of fulfillment that feasting can provide.

During wedding feasts in India, though, food is especially glorious and spiritually symbolic, for it is part of both the nuptials and the ensuing feast. During the nuptials, the food that is "served" into the fire-altar excels as a symbol of transformation as it "ignites" blessings for the couple and contributes to their spiritual union. Afterward, the wedding feast furnishes more spiritual nourishment for the couple, as family and friends celebrate the union with an abundance of blessings and festive food that is "flavored" with the loving emotions inherent in the nuptials.

Feeding the Fire

It is November 18, 1992, in Bombay, India. Indian yoga instructor Nutan Sharma and American physician Arthur Brownstein are marrying at the Gopinath Hindu temple.[6] As each enters the temple separately—first Art, then Nutan—attendants toss flowers and petals in their path. Some guests are seated on the carpet-covered floor just behind the food-laden fire-altar where the couple will exchange vows; others are sitting on chairs, some holding babies; most are talking and laughing and enjoying themselves.

As the ceremony is about to begin, Art stands before the fire-altar, adorned in a white turban and gold-bordered silk *kurta* (a long shirt) over *dhoti,* fine cotton pants. Nutan stands next to him, dressed in a pomegranate-colored silk sari and matching veil, adorned with gold jewelry and fragrant, paisleylike designs drawn in henna on her hands, forearms, and legs. The soft reddish color is a symbol of love and unity. On either side of them are six-foot-high posts decorated with garlands of richly colored flowers. The delicate, soft flowers represent the delicacy of life—the blossoms symbolize a life that blossoms while the various colors signify the ups and downs of life.

Within the square-shaped, clay fire-altar (about two feet square in size), a fire flickers and burns, seemingly reaching toward heaven. According to Hindu tradition, this ritual fire is *Agni,* an ancient Hindu god whose heat is capable of transforming food into consumable meals.[7]

As the fire burns at the center of the clay fire-altar, a cornucopia of seasonal fresh fruit surrounds it: apples, pineapple, grapes, melons, bananas, oranges, and custard apples, representing the fruit of the couple's actions. "When you receive fruits, you offer them back to the Lord," says Pandit Dabral, "and then you are free from past actions. The food also symbolizes the food that will be eaten later on during the feast as a blessing that is shared by everybody."

During the nuptials, the God Agni will consume offerings of various food that the bride and groom present. The fruit that surrounds the fire is there because the fire is believed to be the main witness for the wedding ceremony—the light that is already within the couple, indeed within all of us. Pandit Dabral explained that the *Vedas* consider fire to be the mouth of shining beings called *devas* who live in an invisible, subtle body. Food fed to the *devas* during the marriage ceremony is offered to Agni, so that the food can be transformed into a subtle form that the *devas* can also "consume." In essence, the food is an offering to invisible deities.

Seated on a cushioned mat before the altar-fire, as the pandit (priest) stands on the other side chanting mantras and scripture in Sanskrit, Sharma and Brownstein each place a hand over the other's hand. An attendant wraps a garland of white flowers around their joined hands, tying the floral "rope" into a gentle knot. Then the priest pours water onto the garland.

At this point, instead of exchanging rings as we do in the West, Brownstein presents a *mangal sutra* (literally, "auspicious union") to Sharma by placing it around her neck. Symbolizing their union, it is a gold chain entwined with black beads. As with the wedding ring, the *mangal sutra* announces to the world that Sharma is a married woman.

Now attendants drape a pomegranate-colored cloth across Brownstein's shoulders while joining the other end at Sharma's wrist. After rising while repeating words said by the pandit, Brownstein spoons ghee into the fire, which fuels and inflames it. Representing purity, the ghee is an offering to the *devas* that is "fed" to them in the form of smoke. As with the incense that burns nearby, the smoke ascends toward the heavens.

Then the couple tosses handfuls of puffed rice into the flames, making an offering that represents Sharma's entry into her husband's family. The rice is puffed to symbolize whatever action she has had in her previous family. By tossing the puffed rice into the fire, she is offering herself and her past into it, and making the transition into the new life she is beginning with the new family she will be joining.

Sacred Seven Steps

As the ceremony continues, so too does the melodious Indian music and chanting of the two musicians who are seated on the floor near the fire-altar. At the same time, the pair repeat more sacred words said by the pandit—but this time the words and chants signal the beginning of the seven sacred steps, the essence of the nuptials. Called *saptapadi* in Sanskrit, the steps signify the start of the most important part of the marriage rites. For as the two together walk clockwise around the fruit-laden ceremonial fire seven times, the seventh circling will be recognized as the symbolic moment in which their marriage is sanctified.

As with the rest of the nuptial ceremony, the steps are performed around food—specifically, seven circles of rice that are drawn around the fire. As Brownstein and Sharma perform the circling, they remain joined together by the pomegranate-colored cloth. Reciting special vows from the scriptures during each "round," Sharma begins the first by placing her right foot onto one of the circles of rice.

During each circling, both bride and groom recite meaningful *mantras* (sacred prayers) that confirm their commitment to each other, while expressing what they want out of life. The first one goes like this:

> *Bridegroom*: "My beloved, our love became firm by your walking one step with me. You will offer me the food and be helpful in every way. I will cherish you and provide for the welfare and happiness of you and our children."

> *Bride*: "This is my humble submission to you, my Lord. You kindly give me the responsibility of the home, food, and taking care of the finances. I promise you that I shall discharge all responsibilities for welfare of the family and children."

When Brownstein and Sharma complete the other final seven steps and mantras, they are united as husband and wife. Afterward, they toss more puffed rice into the fire's flickering flames, then, kneeling, each throws in a peeled banana.

Now the nuptials are over, but before the official wedding feast begins, the priest asks the couple to feed each other sweets (a milk-based sweet called *peta*, made from yogurt) to symbolize that they are beginning a new life that will be full of sweetness. It is a sweetness that they will give to each other throughout life from this day forward. Then the feast begins.

Feasting with Family and Friends

"Our wedding feast began in the temple at 11:00 in the morning, right after we were married," says Sharma. "To plan it, my sister, brother, and I sat down two months before the marriage. We decided to have a buffet and caterer for both the first feast, which was for close family and friends, and for the second evening reception, which was for everybody we knew.

"It is written in the *Bhagavad Gita* that when people come to our home, we should be gracious and giving and offer them comfort and love. In Sanskrit, this is called *atithi bava;* it is what food represents in

India. Whenever you go into an Indian home, you will be served something or other—such as sweets or tea. This is the way we greet people.

"We bring this same mentality to the wedding and the food we serve to family and friends. Along with being a gesture of hospitality, sharing food signifies that something auspicious and profound is happening in the family. For when you marry a man in India, you are marrying not only him, but his entire family. To celebrate this, food is always there. It's a way of sharing the commitment with everybody. That's why the wedding feast means something for the whole family, not just for the couple. It is a time to share our joy with the community and relatives.

"After the seven sacred steps around the fire, we began our first wedding feast with about a hundred and fifty close family members and friends. It took place in the same Hindu temple where we were married. During the feast, Arthur and I sat at a special, long table with close family members and special friends that are near and dear to us.

"We ate delicious food from a buffet that included more than a dozen dishes: appetizers such as *papadum,* a round, crispy-thin bread that is made from lentils *(dal);* a variety of breads, such as *puri,* a deep-fried bread filled with vegetables; *paneer makhanwala,* a rich creamy nut sauce with yogurt-like cheese; *pullao,* a rice dish made with saffron, served with an exotic mixture of spiced curry sauce; *samosa,* fried bread stuffed with potatoes and peas; *chutneys,* especially cilantro and pickle; and sweets, including carrot *halva* and *keer,* a rice pudding. Afterward, a refreshing drink, buttermilk *lassi,* was served. This is typically offered after a meal in India, for it is believed to enhance digestion.

"In India, we don't have wedding cake; instead, we serve sweets. If the family can afford it, tradition says that during the marriage feast, there should be five sweets from which to choose. These sweets, which are the richest foods that are served during the ceremony, are the highest expression of hospitality in the Hindu tradition; by making them available to guests, we are showing them the highest regard.

"Most sweets in India contain milk and sugar, fruit, or nuts.

Halva, made from various vegetables such as carrots, squash, and lentils, is typical, and so are *pedas,* which are made from sweetened milk. *Basundi,* a sweet that is made from milk and dried fruit, is cooked for more than five hours until it becomes thick and creamy. When it's finished, it is similar to custard. Another example is *burfee,* a sweet made from milk that is garnished with almonds and other nuts; it is served in little square pieces. *Jelabee,* a delicate pretzel-like sweet, is served warm with syrup.

"Later that evening, we held a reception for more than a thousand people at the Jade Garden in Bombay. Beginning at 6:30 PM, family members and friends came by to offer Arthur and me their blessings, give us a gift, and enjoy the feast. This evening buffet was more elaborate than the one served in the afternoon. There were almost twenty different dishes, which Arthur and I enjoyed after greeting our one thousand guests. The reception ended about 11:00 PM."

Fanciful Five-Day Feast

"Throughout India, different families celebrate weddings differently, often depending on what they can afford. A wealthy friend of mine was married in one of the largest temples in the state of Rajasthan, which means 'the land of the kings.' It is considered to be the most colorful place in India, known for its crafts, especially ceramics. When guests entered this elaborate temple in Rajasthan, camels stood at the entrance to enhance the atmosphere. More than one thousand people attended my friend's wedding feast, which lasted for five days. Rajasthani dancers danced on the stage, and there was much music and singing.

"There were about twenty stalls of food, each consisting of different Rajasthani dishes. People would just walk around, go up to a particular stall and take the food of their choice. Food included typical Rajasthani fare, which means the dishes were somewhat heavy, containing much ghee and hot spices. A typical Rajasthani dish is *kasta katchori,* a crispy fried bread that is stuffed with nuts, *dal,* and many spices; or *ðhehi waða,* a yogurt dish that is served with sweet chutney and *pakoða,* a lentil dish.

"People would eat their food while sitting on the sofas—there were hundreds—that were placed throughout the temple. They also availed themselves of typical Rajasthani crafts—ceramic bangles and clay pots—which were available for the taking at two of the stalls. These were gifts that my friend and her family decided to give to the guests.

"Fifty years ago in India, it was typical for the family itself to prepare the food for the wedding celebration, which would often be attended by hundreds of people in the community. Both men and women would cook in clay pots that were large enough to prepare and hold food for one hundred to two hundred people at a time. They would cook the food over a natural fire made with wood and oil.

"So that guests could eat the food, family members and those in the community would take leaves from a banana tree and use them as plates. To receive the food, hundreds of people would sit in long rows—there may be four rows at one time—while family members would go down the row and serve food to the people on their banana leaves. After the first row had been served, the second row of people would be served, then the third, and so on. After eating, they would throw away the leaves. Then other people would sit down and create another row. So somebody would always be serving and there would always be four or more rows."

Feast of Love

The Hindu marriage ceremony is a rite that both consecrates and purifies the couple through the oblation of food with fire. For most Hindus, the ceremony takes about an hour; for devout Hindus, three hours. Such a rite lies at the core of the Hindu wedding and the ensuing festive feast of elaborate Indian savories. While feasting after a marriage ceremony is a worldwide tradition, what makes the Indian experience particularly unique is the number of celebrants, for in

India it is not unusual for more than one thousand people—relatives, honored guests, and sometimes the entire community—to attend and celebrate the couple's marriage for days on end. "The marriage ceremony is a festival, a big feast in India," says Dabral. "The family invites hundreds of people, and fortunately, as many as you invite, twice as much come. If you invite five hundred, you should prepare for one thousand."[8]

Along with being enjoyed in communion with others, food that is shared at the Hindu wedding feast—and all marriage celebrations—transforms the nuptials and ensuing meal into a sacred act—one that is both an expression of love as well as a connection to the soul. As M. F. K. Fisher wrote, "Food for the soul is a part of all religion.... That is why there can be an equal significance in a sumptuous banquet for five thousand...or in a piece of dry bread eaten alone by a man lifting his eyes unto the hills."[9] And that is why partaking in the wedding feast holds the potential of nourishing both spirit and body—of the bride and groom and all who share their joy and love.

The Spiritual Feast

Because of the spiritual sentiments at its core, the Hindu wedding feast is a manifestation of *bhakti,* a Sanskrit term that means "to eat, partake of, enjoy," as well as "to revere, love."[10] Indeed, the wedding feast, perhaps more than any other celebration, reminds us of the invisible link of love and its ability to bring together family, friends, favorite foods, and festive feelings. In this way, the wedding feast's "very specific rituals and recipes...have the ability to put us in touch with our true feelings about families, nature, and the world around us," writes food journalist Burt Wolf in *Gatherings and Celebrations.*[11]

Based on *bhakti,* the spiritual sensibilities inherent in the Hindu wedding feast, what follows are guidelines for creating your own spiritually centered feast—whether a wedding, New Year celebration, festival, holiday, picnic, barbecue, formal dinner, family meal, or a simple one-course celebration for one. Remember, the essence of a true feast is in the heart and soul of the beholder.

Dine graciously. Appreciate that the food you are enjoying is a gift bestowed by the divine upon humankind. Take pleasure and delight in the abundance, aromas, multicolored hues, textures, and flavors of the food.

Bless the food. To bless food is to honor its life-giving quality. Indeed, early Jewish rabbis believed that eating food without blessing it was to desecrate a holy thing; some believe that the Christian rite of saying grace before a meal has its roots in this tradition.[12] When you are blessed with an abundant feast, and family and friends with whom to enjoy it, take the time to express your appreciation. A simple grace: *Bless this food before me and all those who brought it to my table.*

Connect with life. Enjoying a sumptuous, elaborate meal with others is one of life's greatest pleasures. As you dine, savor the sense of interconnectedness of all life: yourself, family and friends, those who grew, harvested, and prepared the food, and the food itself.

Choose love. Not only is food a loving gift from the divine, Hindus believe that we may present food (or a leaf or flower) as a gift of love to God by offering it "from the heart" in the spirit of true devotion. In this light, the food and drink that is shared at a wedding feast is a form of communal veneration. With each bite, savor this symbiotic relationship.

part two

Psychology,
Science, and
the Spiritual
Ingredient

eleven

Enlightened Eating

A common thread that runs through much research
... is a convergence of science and the ancient wisdom of the spiritual traditions. As it becomes ever
clearer that the area of human consciousness is an
important ... frontier for science and society, we have
to take note of some research laboratories that have
been looking into this matter for thousands of years.[1]

—*Barbara McNeil*

As we have seen throughout this book, turning toward food for
spiritual sustenance is a universal concept that has journeyed through
the centuries, appearing today in every culture and religion throughout the world. Delving into selected ceremonies and customs of various cultures and religions, we have visited the "kitchens" of people
whose spiritual relationship with food is already flourishing.

But this is more than a book about what the wisdom traditions
have to tell us about food's divine essence. It also explores the inter-
section of the wisdom traditions and the scientific world. For, as
researcher David Eisenberg writes, as "we unearth ancient practices,
dust them off ... and study them under the lens of high technology,"
we can "distill simple truths...."[2] By journeying into this neglected
place, the "simple truth" that emerges is that there is more to food
than the biological effects it has on our body.

Spiritual Nourishment

As we have seen, each wisdom tradition has its own way of illuminating food's life-giving qualities: Judaism's concept of holiness espouses approaching food with an appreciative consciousness; Christians commune with the spiritual essence of the divine through the taking of bread and wine during the Eucharist; African Americans invest food with "soul"; yogis turn each encounter with food into an opportunity to experience the "higher" self; Muslims honor food as a blessing from the divine; Buddhists regard food as the nourishment of which enlightened beings partake; Chinese people turn to food to communicate with gods; the Japanese brew tea to nurture spiritual sustenance; Native Americans abstain from food to open themselves to transcendence; and Hindus celebrate weddings with a bountiful food feast—a shared communal meal that is an expression of intermingled blessings and love for the newly married couple.

Indeed, all major religions and traditions speak to a powerful interconnectedness among all life: soil that is nourished through rain, sunshine, and insects; plants that thrive on the elements and photosynthesis; animals that turn to plants for sustenance; and we human beings, who depend on the life forms of plants and food animals for nourishment. In essence, each tradition tells us that by regarding food mindfully, and intentionally bringing a consciousness of gratitude and a loving awareness to our food, we somehow "reintegrate" with the life force in our food, and in so doing are nourished in body and soul.

The spiritual message that emerges when we peel away the layers of the ancient rituals, ceremonies, and traditions that we have been reading about is that all of life is interconnected: the sun, wind, and rain that "fertilizes" food; the soil, plants, and food animals; the many hands who grow and harvest our food; those who bring it to our local grocer; cooks who prepare it; and the family and friends with whom we share our food. In a profound way, we are all "in relationship" to food and with each other.

Intuitively, people from various cultures and religions have turned to food over the centuries as more than sustenance for the body. Instinctively, they knew what researchers are beginning to conjecture: that food is more than simply nourishment for the body, but a potent metaphor for relationship to spirit; that bringing a loving and meditative awareness to food has potentially powerful effects; indeed, when consciously cultivated, such awareness becomes a vehicle for connection to Mother Nature, the Divine, the mystery that is life itself.

Biological Nourishment

Such seemingly metaphysical considerations regarding a symbiotic connection between human consciousness and other life forms are *not* part of the framework of the current biologically oriented nutrition paradigm. This is because traditional nutritional science focuses solely on a biology-based examination of macro- and micronutrients.

Nutritional science has always attempted to understand, explain, or control the contents of our food. It does this by teasing out ever-new information about food's *macro*nutrients — such as protein, carbohydrates, fat, and fiber — as well as its *micro*nutrients, ranging from vitamins and minerals to phytochemicals (naturally occurring substances in plants) and enzymes. This focus on carbohydrates, protein, fat, and fiber, vitamins, minerals, and enzymes, has served us well. It has given us the ability to understand how food affects our health, and prevent and even "reverse" ailments ranging from heart disease to diabetes. But it is an incomplete picture, based on a particular worldview.

The genesis of perceiving food from the perspective of vitamins and minerals goes back to principles of the scientific method developed by Francis Bacon in the 1620s. Other revolutionary scientific discoveries also surfaced in the seventeenth century: William Harvey's insight that the heart circulated blood throughout the body, and Sir Issac Newton's mathematical formulas that could accurately predict the movement of the planets. With these "mechanistic" discoveries, Western civilization started to look at life — including the human body—as something that worked "like a clock," something that could be figured out and predicted—just as the constellations and rotation of the planets could be predicted.

Suddenly big chunks of nature could be explained scientifically with concepts and formulas. European scientists began to believe that humans could have dominion over nature, and that the nature of reality could be explained with the right concepts and formulas. In place of a worldview that had previously been based on superstition and unpredictability, science's new paradigm told us we could measure, predict, and control nature.

Also during this dynamic era, French philosopher René Descartes speculated that our mind (our conscious self) and body (matter) were separate entities—as were our soul and body. Based on these ideas, we came to believe that our consciousness was not connected to nature or any other forms of matter. The result: Our relationship to nature (including our body and mind) became one of separation, alienation, and control. As with the planets and all of nature, our body became material to be measured and controlled, a machine that could be studied independent of mind and soul.

Such a perspective permeated the science of nutrition, which was born in the 1840s when German scientist Justus von Liebig broke foods down into proteins, fats, carbohydrates, and minerals.[3] The calorie, a measure of food energy that French chemist Antoine-Laurent Lavoisier isolated in the eighteenth century,[4] gave us yet another tool with which to measure and control our food intake.

Now, more than a century after these discoveries, nutrition continues to reflect this mechanistic, quantifiable perspective. Not much has changed, for the major focus of biological nutrition continues to be focused on objectifying and measuring what's *in* our food (vitamins, minerals, fat, calories, etc.), and examining how cooking and processing changes the nutrient value of food. With its focus on how the food we eat affects the body, nutrition has become a biological science that dances around the recommended daily allowance (RDA) necessary for optimal health.

Such a perspective is evident in any supermarket you visit. Consider what is written on the package of cereal, bread, milk, or ice cream: the amount of macro- and micronutrients in the food. With a focus on objective numbers and quantities, this is an example of the Newtonian paradigm operating in your everyday food life. It's operating, too, when you count calories, figure the fat grams in your meal, or wonder how much vitamin C you need to combat a cold.

Psychological Nourishment

However, during the past few decades, the focus on what food can do for the body has shifted to what food can do for our mind and emotions. For nutritional science has also begun to explore our psychological and emotional relationship to food through what is often called "food-mood" research. This growing field of mind-body research merges biological nutrition with psychological theories to explore how feelings and emotions affect food choices, and vice versa.

Specifically, it assesses how food affects feelings via hormones (chemical messengers) that are released in the brain when we eat certain foods. The implications: If you become aware of the psychological and emotional dynamics linked to eating, you may be able to choose the food that helps you either relax or think more clearly. And if you become aware of the link between various foods and food cravings, both the cravings and tendency to overeat can be curtailed.

Spiritual Nourishment

While the biological and psychological approaches have been the focus in Western culture, *spiritual* nourishment is at the heart of the new nutritional paradigm I am proposing. Spiritual nourishment explores the *consciousness* that various wisdom traditions suggest we bring to our food, while considering the interrelationship among food-related living entities: the soil, plants, food animals and those who raise them; the friends and family with whom we share our food; and of course, ourselves.

In essence, both the traditional biological and psychological aspects of nutrition emphasize *what food can do for the body*. But the *spiritual* perspective considers another aspect: *what we can do to and for our food,* as well as the influence our thoughts and feelings may have on food. Is it possible that food may receive, store, and "give back" to us the energy and consciousness that we give to our food? This may not be as farfetched as it seems, for we all are aware that through some alchemical process, food becomes life that enters our body and sustains it. Ultimately, food becomes one with us—and we with it—both literally and metaphorically.

The following chapters delve into the psychospiritual research that is just beginning to explore what religionists and spiritualists have hinted at over the centuries: that our thoughts and feelings may influence food—and vice versa. Another dimension that emerges in these chapters is that the food-related beliefs and rituals that we have read about may have evolved from our deep yearning to access and integrate a "perennial wisdom" beyond nourishment for our bodies. Perhaps our deep caring about food and the pleasure we take in food-related rituals emanated from our human spiritual yearning to "digest" love, wisdom, and strength, as well as the energy in our food.

Ultimately, a loving consciousness and the sense of interconnectedness that we bring to food are the threads that weave together ancient food-related wisdom from the spiritual traditions with current scientific theories; they are also the threads that create the fabric of enlightened eating. For enlightened eating acknowledges the inherent sacred quality of food: that it is life-filled and life-giving, offering biological, psychological, and spiritual sustenance.

Let us now join researchers who are studying the various pathways that can lead to enlightened eating. The wisdom that these pathfinders unveil may show us how we may access the sacred significance in food.

twelve

Eating Disorders:
The Starving Spirit

I've come to think that for the person with an eating disorder, hunger becomes...a tangible feeling within the body that matches the inchoate longings of the soul that have no other means of expression: I need, I want, I hunger.[1]

—R. S. Jones

Seeking to help the growing number of people with eating disorders—*anorexia, bulimia,* and **overeating**—the medical community has been striving to understand and treat the causes. Theories abound about why some of us lose control over how much, or little, we eat. Some target cultural influences (the high premium placed on being thin); others consider psychological sources (depression) and biological theories (hormone deficiencies). But there may be yet another more pervasive reason millions of us develop an unhealthy, often life-threatening relationship to food—one that underlies cultural and psychological influences. With food's ability to leave us with a sense of fullness—and its reverse, with emptiness—perhaps eating disorders may result from a "nonspiritual" or disconnected relationship to both the self and food—in other words, the antithesis of the food-related wisdom espoused by world religions and traditions.

The Eating Disorder "Trinity"

Alison's anorexia surfaced when, as a fifteen-year-old high school sophomore, she decided to lose weight. An introvert by nature, she had always wanted to be popular like her pretty, outgoing, thin mother. Finally deciding to do something about it, Alison stopped eating all high-fat food, especially her favorites—ice cream and bread with butter. When she began feeling "lighter" and ethereal, she decided to further slow her eating by cutting all her food—from lettuce to lasagna—into a plethora of tiny pieces, making sure she chewed each piece at least thirty-five times before swallowing. Eventually she limited her daily food intake to only a salad for dinner, but when hunger got the best of her and she ate more than planned, she would exercise to aerobic videos for hours in her room. When her mother finally noticed that her daughter was losing weight, Alison felt elated that she was living up to her mother's standards. What her mother couldn't notice, though, were the bones that were beginning to protrude beneath her daughter's loose-fitting sweaters and skirts. She also remained oblivious to what Alison continued to feel inside: insignificant and unlovable, an asocial failure who was unable to please anyone—especially her mother.

Alison's cousin, Jenny, first exhibited the bingeing and purging symptoms of bulimia when she was twenty years old and a junior in college. Earlier that year Jenny had left home to live in a dormitory on campus. Not too long afterward, she fell in love with Todd, a graduate student teacher in her history class. Her athletic body reflected the many years she had spent in childhood as a competitive gymnast at her parents' urging, yet Jenny had always disliked her body, especially her muscular thighs when she put on extra pounds—as she had now. To "fix" this, she decided to shed eight pounds. Her *modus operandi:* stop munching those muffins and chocolate chip cookies she had always enjoyed when she was alone in her room—away from her parents' ongoing monitoring. When the weight came off, she put on her body-hugging Lycra leotard and "serendipitously" bumped into Todd at the gym where he exercised.

Her strategy worked. Todd noticed her instantly and they dated for almost a year. But when he left her to complete his Ph.D. in Europe, Jenny's emptiness and loneliness became overwhelming. After seeing him off at the airport, she detoured to the local bakery and grocer before returning to her dormitory. In the privacy of her room, she quickly devoured her "mood soother" favorites: four muffins and a bag of her favorite chocolate chip cookies. Then, to regain the sense of control she had lost during the binge, she threw up the food for the first time. For a while she felt relieved, but then the aching emptiness and anxiety returned as she tried to study. Damn, she just couldn't control her compulsion to binge; now she was purging, too.

Eric can't recall *not* having a binge eating disorder (BED), characterized by out-of-control eating *without* purging. His complicated relationship to food manifested when he was quite young. He remembers being only three years old when his mother tried to stop him from climbing on a stool in the kitchen so he could reach the chocolate cookies she had baked that afternoon. All of his memories around food reflect his seemingly endless hunger and his mother's commitment to helping him stay slim. To combat his burgeoning baby fat, his mother began to limit his food—at the pediatrician's suggestion—when he was about four. The food tyranny continued throughout his teens while his mother put him on dozens of diets, ranging from "mostly cottage cheese" to specialized medical plans. Today, at 5'11", Eric weighs almost three hundred pounds. When he tries to limit his food intake, intense feelings of emptiness and worthlessness emerge. So he stopped trying. Instead, he turns to food to feel full. A typical evening food ritual, which usually includes consuming a meal of as much as three thousand calories, leaves him feeling exhausted and "numb." During a typical meal of bacon, eggs, meat, a loaf of bread with butter, cheesecake, cookies, and chocolate, he falls into a stupor; afterward, he drops into a deep, "drugged" sleep.

Alison, Jenny, and Eric each have an eating disorder, defined by psychotherapist Susan Boulware, Ph.D., as "disturbed eating, separating food from the physiological purpose of nourishing the physical body and using it to serve emotional and psychological needs."[2] The "trinity" of eating disorders are: starvation (anorexia nervosa), binging and purging (bulimia), and obsessive overeating (binge eating disorder). Today "among adolescent girls and young women, there is an increasing and disturbing amount of anorexia nervosa and bulimia," writes anorexia historian Joan Jacobs Brumberg in *Fasting Girls: The History of Anorexia Nervosa*.[3] Among men, eating disorders have recently doubled.[4]

"Disturbed Eating" in America

But eating disorders don't only include the "trinity" of anorexia, bulimia, and compulsive overeating. Besides those who have these full-blown disorders are many who hold their cravings in check yet remain preoccupied with food, using it as a way to cope with unpleasant feelings and unresolved problems. Still others are overly concerned about food, hoping to be accepted by a society that demands slimness.

Consider trends in America today: Current research tells us that some girls in the third and fifth grades already worry about fat tummies and thighs and the need to lose weight.[5] Another survey revealed that 50 percent of the women between eighteen and twenty-five years old interviewed preferred to die than be overweight.[6] With our reverence for slimness, a tendency to overeat, fear of fat, and our attraction to magical quick-fix diets, Dr. Boulware and many other health professionals would say most Americans have an undiagnosed eating disorder.

In part, the problem is linked to messages from the media. Americans are constantly bombarded with state-of-the-art "scientific" findings that tell us to avoid fat and keep our weight down. And when we're not reading about the benefits of exercise, leanness, and consuming a low-fat diet, we're watching advertisements and movies that present the ideal female body as being comparable to that of a fourteen-year-old boy. Yet, seemingly oblivious to the message that our food and physical appearance should be lean, restaurants serve portions that are typically double the size of a single "normal" serving. Our food advertisements, too, tell us to eat, eat, eat—a lot, a lot, a lot!

Motivated by the health message but tempted by the pleasures of food, we've taken action by deciding to eat from both corners of our mouths. One side is consuming nonfat foods as never before; for instance, sales of nonfat Snackwell's™ cookies have surpassed those of America's former favorites, high-fat Oreos™ and Chips Ahoy™. Indeed, our daily intake of calories from fat has declined to 34 percent this past decade.[7]

The other side, in the meantime, is enjoying artery-clogging desserts in droves: Ben and Jerry's™ chunky cookie dough ice cream is the company's best-seller; Häagen-Dazs™ ice cream sales are booming, too.[8] Throwing caution to the wind, we're eating more and gaining more. A 1994 survey by the United States Department of Agriculture (USDA) revealed that about one-third of us are overweight, and the average person weighs eleven to twelve pounds more than they did in the late 70s.[9] Concerned about our tendency to put on pounds, researcher John Foreyt, Ph.D., of the Baylor College of Medicine, predicted in the medical journal Lancet that by the year 2230, if our weight-gain trend continues, 100 percent of American adults will be overweight.[10]

But while there may be a culture-wide obsession about fat, food, optimal nutrition, and "being thin," what is it that causes eight million Americans—about one in ten male[11]—to "cross over" from irrational eating and thinking about food into a full-blown eating disorder?

Many believe the answer to "disturbed eating" is multicausal: a culture obsessed with being thin, unexpressed emotional problems, and/or a genetic predisposition to depression. But these cultural, psychological, and biological theories only partially explain eating disorders. Perhaps the cause lies elsewhere—in a culturally nurtured spiritual starvation that permeates many aspects of our lives.

Cultural Cues

"The symptoms of disease never exist in a cultural vacuum," writes Jean Brumberg.[12] The reasons for our culture's ambivalent relationship to food—and ensuing eating disorders—are numerous, but psychologist David Riesman expressed the underlying cultural causes most eloquently in his classic book *The Lonely Crowd*.[13] According to Riesman, America went from being "inner directed" in the nineteenth century, to twentieth-century values that encompass "outer-directedness" and a focus on external image rather than internal cues.

Consider life in the nineteenth century, when people were guided by a set of stable, time-honored, unquestioned, internalized religious and moral codes or ideals, such as integrity, kindness, and generosity. Most people lived in small towns and rural communities where these values were reinforced by family, friends, religion, and community. Living from this set of internal values and feelings, they felt connected to others, and experienced a sense of belonging.

By the twentieth century, life had changed. Today most of us live in or near urban centers, often far from our families, with little connection to our communities. As science replaced religion as our higher "authority," success in life no longer means being guided by our internal values and the well-being of our community; rather, the criteria has shifted to external standards and a focus on the self, especially the image we present to the world: our accomplishments, prestige, the clothes we wear, our cars and homes—and how thin and attractive we are. In the process, as we learned to pursue images for fulfillment, we lost touch with our inner essence, our true selves. Explains clinical psychologist Michael Mayer, Ph.D., "When we allow the craving for external images, such as being thin or looking perfect, to replace our more essential needs, such as our need for love, connectedness, learning, and right livelihood, then we become addicted to the sweets of life, rather than to the main meal, where true nourishment lies."[14]

Some have rebelled against our cultural worship of thinness, such as members of *About-Face*, a San Francisco-based group that launched the "Stop Starvation Imagery Campaign." Its satirical poster shows ultrathin model Kate Moss in the nude with the words "Emaciation Stinks" above her bone-thin body; the words "Stop Starvation Imagery" frame the bottom section of the poster. Still others have joined a "big is beautiful" campaign in an attempt to accept their bodies, regardless of size.

But these groups are the exception, not the rule. For in a self-involved, outer-directed culture, the image we present to society is all-important. But for many of us, pursuing such an image is destined to fail because an image, like a mirage, is unreal and mercurial, external and artificial. The result: unable to achieve a superficial, unrealistic goal, our sense of insecurity and anxiety grows—along with a need for control through perfectionism. And all the while, our inner essence, our soul, remains ignored, bypassed, unregarded, unseen—starved.

When Image is All

The classic Greek myth of Narcissus epitomizes the heartfelt damage that is inflicted when either society, or an individual, is not regarded. When the goddess Juno suspected her husband was amusing himself with the wood nymphs, Echo, one of the beautiful but talkative nymph, diverted Juno's attention so that the other nymphs would have time to escape. Discovering the manipulation, Juno punished Echo by limiting her power of speech to repeating the last syllable of words she heard from others. Later, when Echo fell in love with the handsome youth Narcissus, she could not communicate with him until he spoke to her. But when he did, though she tried to speak to him with all her heart, all she could do was repeat the last word he had uttered.

Abruptly spurned by Narcissus and feeling thoroughly rejected by him, Echo died of a broken heart. When the gods learned of Narcissus' callousness, they vowed he would live only until he saw his own reflection. One day when he beheld his image in the waters of a fountain, he fell passionately in love. Refusing to leave his reflection, he remained at the fountain until he died and became the narcissus flower.

The myth of Narcissus personifies the dilemma we create for ourselves when we pursue an image. "Falling in love with one's image — that is, becoming narcissistic—is seen in the myth as a form of punishment for being incapable of loving," explains Alexander Lowen, M.D., in *Narcissism: Denial of the True Self*.[15] But what about Echo? She suffered by living her life as a reflection of others' words. Ultimately, Narcissus' inability to love her (or anything but his own image, for that matter) led her to die of a broken heart.

Is it possible that those with eating disorders—and the millions of us who are overconcerned and preoccupied with food—suffer as Echo did? Could it be that they turn to food to fill the void of not having been loved by someone who, ultimately, cannot truly love; by someone (or some "thing," such as our culture) who is more interested in her or his own image than another person? Could it be that self-involvement as well as our image-obsessed culture conspire together to create a spiritual void and loss of self in those who strive to be loved and accepted by those who are incapable of loving?

Psychologist Carl Rogers believes so. "In order to receive approval and love, [sometimes] we learn to suppress those feelings and expressions of ourselves that are deemed unacceptable to the important caretakers in our lives," he writes. Over time, we no longer "recognize the difference between what is internal [our real needs and feelings] and...external [the needs of another], to know who we really are."[16] The result? We lose touch with the "wisdom of [our] organism,"[17] no longer knowing what we think or feel. Having surrendered our true self and needs, we become self-starved.

Delve into the personal stories and psychological profiles of people with eating disorders and certain painful emotional states continually emerge: Victims grope to express the inexpressible with words such as "empty," "low self-esteem," "unworthy," "depressed," "unlovable"; many talk of "servicing" others' needs while ignoring their own. Witness Princess Diana describing the feelings that motivated her bouts with bulimia, on ABC News' *Turning Point:* "I'd come home and it would be very difficult to know how to comfort myself, having been comforting lots of other people. So it would be a regular pattern to jump into the fridge.... You inflict it [bulimia] on yourself because your self-esteem is at a low ebb and you don't think you're worthy or valuable. You fill your stomach up four or five times a day...and it gives you a feeling of comfort. It's like having a pair of arms around you, but it's temporary—temporary."[18]

There are many psychological theories that explain how or why such eating disorders occur, but the most penetrating includes the devastating effects that narcissistic, self-involved parents, often the mother, can have on a child. In *The Drama of the Gifted Child*, Alice Miller tells us that if a mother is emotionally insecure, she is often unresponsive or unaware of her child's real needs. In turn, the child is "trained" to conform to the frequently self-aggrandizing, image-oriented needs of the mother, long before he or she is consciously capable of doing so. The result: the child's needs for authentic inter-action, respect, admiration, mirroring, and unconditional regard go unmet.[19]

As with Echo, underlying these painful feelings is the sense of being rejected and unloved for herself. Having accepted the "reflec-tion" from another that she is unworthy, a deep sense of sadness and emptiness emerges. To cope with such deep spiritual despair, some turn to food for comfort, to numb the unrelenting emotional pain; oth-ers may internalize the core rejection of their self with a sense of worthlessness, believing they are not even significant enough to live— as is the case with some anorexics.

After successfully battling her own eating disorder, therapist Melody Marks, M.S.W., concluded that "the beginning of an addic-tion occurs the moment the child feels he or she is not lovable, is not loved.... And the pain of that experience, of that knowledge...is what one wants to numb oneself from, or get away from."[20]

Dr. Boulware agrees: "Without love, the spirit suffers. The child grows up thinking she must be wrong, there's something wrong with her or him. Ultimately, an inner voice or 'critic' develops, which can literally kill the child in the form of suicide but, more typically, it takes the form of other destructive behaviors: substance abuse, overwork, abusive relationships. When the addiction is food, it becomes a concrete symbol of some spiritual nourishment that's needed. The impulse isn't wrong; in fact, it's healthy. But the method by which the person chooses to satisfy it will inevitably be very self-destructive."[21]

Spiritual Sustenance

Turning around the self-destructive impulses linked to eating disorders isn't easy, but we now know that when victims of eating disorders are given unconditional love (caring for a person for who she is "inside"—regardless of "external" behavior and appearance), it is possible for them to make the journey from inner torment to recovery.

When her own children were starving from anorexia, Canadian psychologist Peggy Claude-Pierre knew she had to do something immediately if her two daughters were to survive. The signs of anorexia first surfaced in Kirsten, her then-fifteen-year-old daughter. It was at a time when Claude-Pierre was separated from her first husband and working on her doctorate in psychology.

Concerned and receiving inadequate help from the medical community, Claude-Pierre realized she needed to understand the psychology of the disorder if she was to help her daughter. In response, she stayed by Kirsten's side for a year and a half, observing everything she did. Soon Claude-Pierre learned to "hear" and understand the inner voices (common to those with eating disorders) that constantly told her daughter she was unlovable and not even worthy enough to eat. She learned that "they go into their head to listen to the voices that are putting them down."[22]

Realizing that a lack of self-respect and self-worth—a starving spirit—and a distorted self-image was behind everything her daughter said, did, and heard from the inner voices, Claude-Pierre figured out the only possible solution: unrelenting unconditional love. But then as Kirsten began healing, her thirteen-year-old sister Nicole also became anorexic. Over time, though, Claude-Pierre's unconditional love healed Nicole's anorexia, too.

Today, both daughters are healthy, "normal" eaters, with no concern about recidivism. As a matter of fact, they now help other victims of eating disorders at their mother's Montreux Counseling Center in Victoria, Canada. Here, Claude-Pierre's treatment of ongoing, unlimited, unconditional love has been doing the impossible: turning around victims of eating disorders who are on the verge of death. And breaking tradition with a disease that has only a 50 percent recovery rate (and from which 20 percent of chronic sufferers die),[23] those who complete the center's program seem to recover without a later relapse.[24]

For many suffering from eating disorders, there is a sense of not having been cared for in the way they needed to be. What remains is a sense of "dis-connection," a spiritual deficit that locks them into the illusion of being unworthy; feeling unworthy, they are uncomfortable with, and resistant to, accepting love. This is exemplified by a comment made by one of Claude-Pierre's patients: "They showed you so much love [at the center] and I hated them for it.... I didn't want them to love me. Well, I suppose I did, deep down, but I...didn't want to accept it. I didn't think I should."[25]

Until Claude-Pierre's work, many perceived anorexia as a compulsion to lose weight. But we now know that "voices" in the victims' minds are telling them that they don't deserve to eat, to live—or to be loved. Says Claude-Pierre: "It's voices telling them that they're unworthy and directing them to hurt themselves. These kids have a broken spirit, broken identity.... They don't think they deserve to live. It's not that they don't want to. Everybody wants to live if they know how...They need a map, to be shown."[26]

The Transformative Power of Love

What is it about Peggy Claude-Pierre's "map" and authentic, unconditional love that is capable of restoring the spirit and will to live? How is she able listen to inner voices, changing a person bent on self-destruction into one filled with self-acceptance and self-love, able to embrace life?

Addiction therapist Jacquelyn Small, M.S.S.W., would say Claude-Pierre works her magic because she is a "transformer," a person who "is here to remind us of our Essence...the Self we were intended to be before we lost our way."[27] With penetrating kindness and insight, transformers see through our facades, helping us to face our addictions and connect with our true selves with dignity and authenticity.

They "work with what *is* about us, not what 'ought to be' by someone else's standards," explains Small. "And by their positive acceptance of us—their total endorsement of our being—they serve as catalysts...to weed out the *im*perfection, focusing on clearing the way for more and more of the authentic masterpiece to shine through."[28] In short, they give people unconditional love, helping them to transform themselves into who they really are.

Through Claude-Pierre's ability to help those with eating disorders transform—when people prone to this problem are nourished with love—we are offered a glimpse into the human spirit's ability to rejuvenate and heal. But along with depending on others (such as a good therapist, support group, friends, or loving family members) to heal, those with eating disorders can become their own "transformers," capable of using their own loving energy to change an eating disorder-laden life into one that is eating disorder-free, spiritually rich, sustaining, and soul-satisfying.

To achieve such transcendence, though, calls for a willingness to leave an emotional space that is familiar and comfortable, though it does not feel good, nor is good for you. For many, it means changing the belief that tells you that if you're thin, you will be loved. It calls for the willingness to listen to what your inner voices are telling you; to remain open to accepting all emotions that may surface. It calls for the realization that feelings are signals, clues that can give you answers and insights into the work you must be willing to do in order to leave the tyranny of food addiction.

The Road Back

The journey to "the other side" of an eating disorder calls for coming to terms with the past and forgiving ourselves and others. It challenges us to view our addiction to food as something we thought we needed to help us through painful feelings—although it was the wrong kind of help. It asks us to view our eating disorder as a spiritual teacher that can lead us to our true essence. Says Small: "For the addicted, awareness and a willingness to work on oneself provide the springboard for this inward, upward journey that takes us first into ourselves and finally beyond ourselves."[29]

What follows is a brief look into ways others have transcended eating disorders, either their own or by helping others overcome theirs. The common thread: achieving transcendence through a connection with love, God, a Higher Being, the Ultimate. Only through this connection can those who suffer from eating disorders find the peace and connection to the themselves they had lost years before.

Jo Ind's Story

"When I was a compulsive eater it was not just my pain that I was cutting off from, it was God-in-me too," writes Jo Ind in *Fat is a Spiritual Issue: My Journey*, describing the ongoing spiritual emptiness that drove her to fill it with food.[30] When Ind decided she no longer wanted to binge and overeat to fill her spiritual void, she began by listening to and changing her self-talk. Instead of feeling self-contempt after a binge and vowing to start dieting, she focused on getting in touch with her lost appetite and feelings. Here is a brief explanation about the beginning of her transformation, excerpted from her book:

"I learnt to retrace my appetite by asking myself, 'Am I hungry?' and [if I was] then eating whatever I wanted. I learnt to retrace my feelings by giving myself space to experience them whenever I felt the urge to smother them in doughnuts. 'Am I hungry?' No. So why do I want to eat? Am I worried? Am I afraid? Am I guilty? What's going on in this life of mine? Is my heart hurting? What are my guts groaning? God you are in me. What are you saying?"[31]

By persevering, over time she was able to access her "deepest place, the seat of my passions, and [let] them permeate the rest of my being."[32] For Ind, by "allowing God-in-me to be,"[33] she was able to use love to connect her psyche (everyday consciousness, thoughts, and feelings) and soul (the eternal part of our Self that is incapable of suffering, dieting, starving, or dying), no longer needing to turn to food for sustenance.

Leonard Laskow's Techniques

Another approach for "releasing" eating disorders is through what Leonard Laskow, M.D., calls *holoenergetic healing*. In his book *Healing with Love*, Dr. Laskow describes his model "based on expanded awareness, love, and the empowerment that comes from making a conscious choice for change. Once you are certain you are willing to 'transform,'" he says, "begin by recognizing or locating what is currently 'in form' that you want to change."[34]

Dr. Laskow's techniques give readers the tools to "harness" spiritual energy and transform it into loving, healing energy. Here is the essence of his healing techniques, modified to address eating disorders.

Intention: Identify your positive intention, what it is you want to change. This is an inner want that you can see or feel; it is not actions and goals. For instance, deciding to eat healthful foods is an intention; losing weight, a goal.

Visualization. When you're not hungry but are feeling an urge to eat, envision (fantasize, daydream) what you might do instead to obtain a sense of self-love. Some options: call up a good friend, take a warm bubble bath, or meditate in a favorite room.

Love. Experiencing unconditional love means accepting yourself for who you are, not for what you want to be or look like. After you identify your behavior and practice positive visualization, fill your being with compassion and caring for your mind, body—even your eating disorder.

The Love-Powered Diet

Victoria Moran got off the roller-coaster of destructive eating habits by learning how to nourish herself from within. In her book *The Love-Powered Diet: A Revolutionary Approach to Healthy Eating and Recovery from Food Addiction,* she says that we must connect "with our spiritual selves, by making practical contact with the Divine, whatever we perceive that to be."[35]

Convinced that eating disorders are due to a "spiritual hunger," Moran suggests feeding ourselves with "spiritual food."[36] Although her approach is extensive, here is a sampling of her "revolutionary concepts" designed to change your relationship to both your body and food. She suggests meditating on one or more of these spiritually oriented concepts both in the morning and evening.

- *Food addiction is serious and, like other addictions, progressive. Few genuine addicts have ever recovered without a spiritual basis.* Consider that relating to something "larger" than yourself creates a source of fulfillment other than food. Therefore, developing a spiritual link can improve the odds of recovery.

- *You are a spiritual being living in a physical body. Your body is an integral part of the totality that is you.* Consider that true joy and fulfillment come from satisfying your spiritual essence, rather than your physical body.

- *Your body is not an independent entity; it reflects what's going on inside you—emotionally, mentally, and spiritually.* Consider that you are more—much more—than your body. When your emotions and spiritual essence are in sync, this unity is likely to manifest itself in a more balanced relationship to food.[37]

The Wisdom Within

There are a multitude of ways to access the wisdom within our souls, ultimately creating a loving relationship to food and ourselves. Just as each person has a unique set of circumstances that leads to an eating disorder, so too are there various ways to bring authentic love into your life. Along with the insights of those discussed in this chapter who have learned to use love to move beyond eating disorders, we have seen throughout this book how various people from diverse cultures and religions have created their own ways of "digesting" love and wisdom from the food they prepare and eat.

When we are willing to listen to the wisdom of our bodies and release our eating disorders into the healing light of love, we give ourselves a chance to transform the spiritual starvation in our hearts and souls, while learning to feed ourselves life's optimal nourishment: love. The benefits of such a gift to ourselves are limitless. For eating disorders are not only about the food we turn to for bodily nourishment, they are driven by a deeper, instinctive understanding that "hearts starve as well as bodies; give us bread but give us roses."[38]

Transformation Techniques

A close look at the spiritual and emotional worlds of those who have transcended their eating problem reveals many similarities. They each realized that learning to love and transform themselves wasn't easy, but that it was possible, with much patience and commitment. Over time, instead of turning to others and food for the "answer," they learned to connect to their true selves. This meant regarding themselves for who they are, seeing themselves for who they are, and accepting themselves for who they are—in short, loving themselves.

As you come to understand the insights that follow, keep in mind that the most important ingredients are *you*, your own thoughts, feelings, insights, and your willingness to embrace and appreciate the process of becoming who and what you already are. Regardless of whether or not you have an eating disorder, the following suggestions, which may spark insights that will help you to stop starving yourself of your Self, are just the beginning of this lifetime journey. To begin:

Identify the behavior you want to change, then decide to *intend* (rather than wish or hope) to do something about it. By identifying specifically what it is you want to change, you're clarifying your goal. For instance, you may want to stop overeating (the behavior you want to change) and become a person who eats *only* when you are hungry, and stopping when full instead of stuffed (your intention, aim, or purpose).

Listen to your inner voice(s) so you can identify the true feelings, needs, and wants behind your food issues. To begin, consider keeping a journal. Whenever you're overcome with the urge to eat—or *not* eat even though you're hungry—identify and write down what it is you were thinking, feeling, or doing when the urge surfaced. For example, perhaps the urge to splurge—or avoid food—intensifies whenever you come home from school or work and you're alone. If so, ask yourself which feelings are percolating beneath the surface at that time. Anxiety? Loneliness? Depression? Panic? Sadness?

If it's hard for you to identify feelings, consider asking yourself what happened during the day. Did you feel socially inept? Arrive late for a meeting? Perhaps nothing specific happened, but you're anxious anyway. Whatever surfaces, write it down. By identifying your thoughts and feelings, you are really listening to the inner voices that lead you to eat or not eat. Writing down what you "hear" can help you develop a more focused picture of the situations and feelings that are linked with your eating problem.

Take charge by talking back to your negative inner voices, feelings, and thoughts. If they're pushing you to do something you no longer want to do, tell them! If they're telling you to feel something you don't want to feel, let them know! If they're telling you to buy that bag of your favorite muffins, shout No way!—loudly. If they're repeating that you're worthless and fat, fight back. Tell them, That's not true! with conviction. A brief, direct No! or Stop! can be effective too.

Act on what you want to change by envisioning the new behavior. Inhaling deeply to relax, try closing your eyes and visualizing coming home after work or school. Imagine feeling lonely, then hearing your inner voice telling you to eat a bag of blueberry muffins to relieve the emptiness. Now's the time to talk back to your voice. Tell it you're no longer willing to respond blindly to its orders anymore. Then consider telling it you don't need it anymore. But first, thank your voices for what they've been trying to do for you all these years (protect you from painful feelings). Then say good-bye and let...them...go.

Another way to begin acting on what you want to change is by imagining what you would do instead of eating: take a walk at dusk, call a good friend, read a book, look at the sky, listen to the rain.

Love your Self by appreciating and *being* with yourself, instead of *doing* what self-destructive voices are dictating. You're choosing self-love when you speak to yourself with care and concern rather than judgment and anger, take a walk instead of a cookie, stop eating because your body has told you it's had enough, or "de-stress" by meditating instead of munching on that muffin. In short, you are finding pleasure in *being* with yourself, rather than turning to food to avoid it.

thirteen

The Food-Mood Connection

According to ancient texts...venerable
scientists...discovered...that food is an embodiment of the life-force; it affects us on all levels—
physical, mental, emotional, and spiritual.[1]
—Carrie Angus, M.D.

With all that we now know about the
food/mind/mood connection...you can begin to
select [food] that will...modify your moods
and...make you a more effective, motivated, and
perhaps even more contented individual.[2]
—Judith Wurtman, Ph.D.

As we have seen in Chapter 5, for centuries yogis have eaten certain foods for their psychological effects. In China, too, food has been used for thousands of years to calm and focus the mind. What follows is a look into the modern science that is discovering what ancient spiritual seekers learned intuitively: that foods release substances in our bodies that effect our emotions and moods.

Often called food-mood research, this emerging science offers new insights into our spiritual well-being. It encourages us to regard food for its effects on our body-mind. At the same time, it helps us to recognize and appreciate that the relationship between food and our emotions is yet another key ingredient to enlightened eating.

Calming Calories

Imagine choosing one type of food to alleviate anxiety, another to bolster brainpower, yet another to curb your urge to splurge on that donut. You can accomplish this—and more—by eating specific foods throughout the day. A new field of pioneering nutrition research, often referred to as the study of food and mood, is confirming what many have always suspected: what and when we eat can affect our mind and mood, our tendency to pile on pounds, even the quality of our lives.

Richard Wurtman, M.D., and Judith Wurtman, Ph.D., scientists at the Massachusetts Institute of Technology (MIT), first linked food with mood when they found that the sugar and starch in carbohydrate foods boosted a powerful brain chemical called serotonin.[3] Soon they linked serotonin and other neurotransmitters (substances that pass information from cell to cell in the brain) to our every mood, emotion, or craving. For instance, they noted that eating a carbohydrate-rich food, such as grains, beans and peas, and vegetables, elevated serotonin levels, helping you to feel more relaxed and calm; high-protein foods, such as dairy products, fish, poultry, and meat, had the opposite effect: they released substances that let you think and react more quickly and feel more alert and energetic.

Carbohydrate Cravings

It might be easy to interpret food-mood research to mean that athletes shouldn't eat carbohydrates before competing because they'll be too relaxed to perform well. "This isn't true," says Catherine Christie, Ph.D., R.D., nutritionist and author of *I'd Kill For a Cookie*. "When you look at the recommendations for carbohydrates in athletes, whenever they participate in an athletic event, the adrenaline that's associated with competition seems to override any of the other effects that would be associated with serotonin and relaxation." To eat to win, "we recommend a carbohydrate diet because it is the body's preferred fuel, and adults do better with endurance exercise when they eat a high-carbohydrate diet."

More current studies have shed additional light on issues surrounding carbohydrate intake and mood. Researchers at Rockefeller University in New York believe food cravings may be Mother Nature's way of informing women what they need to eat to feel better. Perhaps sugar cravings many women experience at puberty, premenstrually, during pregnancy, and after menopause could be a response to estrogen's effect on brain chemicals and blood sugar levels.

"Women may be more sensitive to changes in serotonin than men," explained Dr. Christie when she talked with me on the phone from her office in Jacksonville, Florida. "When estrogen levels fall and progesterone levels are high, serotonin levels may drop. We postulate that this drop is why women crave carbohydrates during certain times of the menstrual cycle. If serotonin levels fall, appetite increases, particularly for carbohydrates." The same mechanism seems to occur during menopause. "When estrogen levels decline," she says, "there's often increased appetite, carbohydrate craving, and reported weight gain. This may also be related to changes in serotonin."[4]

Fat, Mood and Memory

Taking the female food/mood research a step further, University of Michigan researchers have linked the desire for sugar with its ability to calm; for fat, with its ability to elevate moods. Adam Drewnowski, Ph.D., director of the Human Nutrition Program at the University of Michigan, believes it's not carbohydrates women crave, it's fat. The real craving, he thinks, is triggered when we combine sugar with fat, creating a sweet-and-creamy concoction that's hard to resist. According to Drewnowski and Barbara Smith, Ph.D., a researcher at Johns Hopkins University in Baltimore, it is really the *endorphins*, naturally occurring substances in the brain that function as painkillers and produce pleasurable feelings, that we're really after when we go after a Dove Bar™. They believe we crave high-fat, sugar-laden foods to experience the blues-busting benefits of endorphins. These findings could explain why many women crave chocolate. With its half fat/half sugar content, chocolate may offer the perfect blend of ingredients both to stimulate and soothe at the same time.[5]

"Chocolate also contains phenylethylamine (PEA)," says Dr. Christie, "a substance that is thought to enhance endorphin release." Not only is PEA released when we eat chocolate, it also produces its euphoric side effects when we fall in love.

Does understanding why we crave chocolate give us carte blanche to reach for chocolate whenever the craving strikes? Yes, in small amounts, believes Debra Waterhouse, M.P.H., R.D., author of *Why Women Need Chocolate: Eat What You Crave to Look and Feel Great*.[6] She recommends avoiding high-fat, sugar-laden foods most of the time. But when a craving for chocolate or other food strikes, surprisingly small amounts can balance brain chemistry and moods. Waterhouse believes that women's biological cravings aren't a problem to be overcome, but a signal about what our bodies need. Ironically, suppressing the craving instead of allowing an occasional indulgence can lead to overeating and weight gain.

While the fat and sugar in chocolate may explain why many women turn to it as a soothing "friend," it helps to know that not all fat has been created equal. Animal fat in particular may dim memory and mental abilities. "Rats fed lard cannot find their way through mazes as easily as rats fed soybean oil," writes Jean Carper in *Food—Your Miracle Medicine*. "The biggest culprit...is saturated-type animal fat."[7]

Anti-Stress Strategies

Though many women instinctively choose chocolate to modify mood, another nutritional strategy may work to ease stress-related tension. When United States Department of Agriculture researchers studied the physical and emotional impact a high-stress week had on people eating adequate diets, they found that blood and tissue levels of certain vitamins and minerals dropped by as much as 33 percent. In the long-term, this depleted nutrient supply can translate into a weakened immune system and lowered resistance to ailments ranging from colds and infections to cardiovascular disease, asthma, and perhaps cancer, concludes Elizabeth Somer in her book *Food and Mood*.[8] The remedy? She suggests a plethora of vitamins and minerals that are especially vital to nourishing the body when it's under stress, including magnesium, antioxidants (especially C, E, and beta-carotene), and B vitamins.

Somer also recommends "keeping away from the two worst offenders: caffeine [found in chocolate, coffee, tea, and cola] and refined sugar." Her rationale: "During times when you need your mental, physical, and emotional reserves, sugar and caffeine can send your blood-sugar levels plummeting and leave your brain chemistry in disarray."[9]

To ease stress, Somer suggests avoiding caffeine and alcohol as well as high-fat, high-sugar, low-nutrient sweets. Instead, choose high-fiber foods (fruits, vegetables, whole grains, legumes). And if stress overload has caused you to lose your appetite, eat small meals throughout the day.

The Caffeine Kick

Caffeine. It's used by millions of people to feel better and "get through the day." It's a psychoactive drug that can lift your mood and make you more mentally alert. Too much can trigger anxiety, panic attacks, and insomnia; too little for the "addicted" is likely to bring withdrawal symptoms ranging from headaches to depression and fatigue. Closer scrutiny by scientists of this popular drug has revealed that caffeine is a paradoxical substance. It works its wonders by suppressing what former CNN medical correspondent Jean Carper calls "'down' brain chemicals instead of releasing 'up' chemicals. [This causes] brain cells [to] remain in a state of excitability," she explains in *Food — Your Miracle Medicine*.[10]

How much caffeine is enough to produce mental alertness? As little as a cup or two of coffee (100-200 mg.) daily or a small serving of carbonated cola (32 mg.) can improve mental performance and alertness, reduce fatigue, and work as a natural antidote to the slump many of us experience after eating. But when it comes to caffeine, more isn't necessarily better. Caffeine abuse can produce anxiety, restlessness, and other symptoms ranging from traumas and headache to irregular heartbeat, elevated blood pressure and cholesterol, nutrient deficiencies, and poor concentration.[11]

For those who have an addiction, "detoxing" from caffeine can be just as unpleasant. Withdrawal symptoms can include headaches, irritability, depression, fatigue, nausea, and cramps. As with most nutritional recommendations, moderation seems to be the key to success.

Which Comes First, Food or Mood?

While most researchers agree that a physiological "switch" occurs when we eat certain foods, not all agree on the cause. Why? Because the chemical cornucopia in our brains and bodies isn't always easy to understand. In the world of science, it's hard to establish a direct link between our brain chemistry and our physical or emotional response. This is because our predisposition for some foods could be based on previous conditioning that links positive feelings with that food. For instance, if your mother rewarded you with chocolate chip cookies for doing well in school, you may continue to reward yourself with cookies as an adult when you finish a challenging task. Or perhaps choosing certain foods may not be about mood, but about what your body must have to meet its nutrient needs; this may mean you choose to snack on an orange for its vitamin C content, not its food-mood affect. Or perhaps feelings drive you to choose certain foods: a piece of pie may alleviate boredom; crunching on carrots or celery could augment anger. Because the interaction is so complex, food-mood research is still in its infancy.

Designing Moods

Given what science has currently revealed, what information is practical to use in our everyday lives? Dr. Christie believes that every person's situation is different. "People who have had a real stressful day
may want to consider a carbohydrate snack—perhaps air-popped
popcorn—in the afternoon to help them relax a bit. However, if they
have a super-important meeting at 4:00 PM, it may make more sense
to choose a high-protein snack, such as nonfat yogurt, to get more of
an alertness effect."

The interplay among people, brain chemistry, and food is complex: not all food will affect everyone the same way. For instance,
while high-carbohydrate foods produce a calming affect in most people, they seem to stimulate and energize those who experience pre-
menstrual syndrome (PMS) or the winter depression of Seasonal
Affective Disorder (SAD), says Carper.[12] Regardless, if we choose
our food consciously, it holds the potential to recharge, sustain, and
nurture our emotions and moods.

With this in mind, here are some of Carper's mood-food suggestions, detailed in her book *Food—Your Miracle Medicine:*

Energy-enhancers. Protein-rich foods: low-fat seafood, turkey breast,
nonfat milk, lowfat or nonfat yogurt, coffee; boron-containing foods
such as fruits, nuts, legumes, broccoli, apples, pears, peaches, grapes.

Memory-boosters. Thiamin-containing foods: wheat germ, bran, nuts,
fortified cereal, meat; riboflavin-containing foods: almonds, fortified
cereals, milk, liver; carotene-containing foods: dark green, leafy vegetables, orange fruits and vegetables; zinc-rich foods: seafood;
legumes, cereals, whole grains.

Blues busters. Beans, pasta, vegetables, cereal, bread, crackers,
sweets; folic acid-containing foods: spinach and other dark, leafy
greens, lima beans; selenium-containing foods: brazil nuts, canned
light tuna, cooked oysters, sunflower seeds, puffed wheat cereal,
swordfish or clams, garlic, chili peppers (which contain capsaicin).

Anxiety alleviators. Complex carbohydrates, especially potatoes, pasta, bread, beans and cereal, onions; snacks: honey or sugar, low-fat, high-carbohydrate foods such as air-popped popcorn, rice cakes, Cheerios™, and other dry breakfast cereals. Avoid caffeine-containing beverages (coffee, black and green tea, colas, chocolate), especially if they are not a part of your usual diet—sudden caffeine consumption can make you nervous and anxious. Avoid alcohol.

Memory-dimmers. Saturated animal fat: lard, butter, high-fat meat, poultry, fish, cheese and other dairy; alcohol.[13]

When considering which foods to eat when, the first consideration is: do no harm. If a food-mood recommendation will ultimately limit, or conflict with your preferred diet, then the particular food may not be appropriate for you. When evaluating food-mood recommendations, ask yourself, Is this something that's reasonable for me to eat, to include in my diet? After considering the potential benefits of certain foods, consider your personal food preferences. The goal is to become aware of the gentle message in your meals, to use your food choices to gain more control over your moods, and in the process, enhance spiritual well-being.

Savoring Food and Feelings

Ultimately, food-mood research is an investigation of food and how the mind and body work together. By being aware of this connection, food offers us an opportunity to pay attention to, and connect with, our body-mind. Seen in this light, each food we choose to eat may be looked at as an opportunity not only to feed the body but also to "fine-tune" our moods and emotions. And as it does, food becomes a path to self-understanding, a tool for exploring the Self.

When we select food mindfully—with an awareness of our state of mind and how food may affect it—food carries the potential of letting us "digest" a sense of order, harmony, and well-being. Ultimately, by holding the potential to nurture our feelings and moods, food may bring us a step closer to accessing our spiritual Self. If we pause to regard, to sense, and to savor the effects of food, we may also catch a glimpse of its ability to both nurture and transform us—ever so gently.

Eating to Enhance Emotions

Based on Judith Wurtman's book *Managing Your Mind and Mood Through Food*, here are some food-mood suggestions for enhancing emotions from morning to night.

Breakfast. ½ grapefruit or 4 ounces fruit juice; 1 cup plain yogurt; ½ cup low-fat granola.
Nutrient capsule: Low fat, high carbohydrate, high protein, nutrient-dense.
Food-mood strategy: Calms and energizes.

Mid-morning snack. Whole-grain, low-fat crackers; low-fat milk.
Nutrient capsule: High protein, high carbohydrate.
Food-mood strategy: Calms and energizes.

Business lunch. Chef's salad made with 1½ cups salad greens; fat-free dressing; 1 ounce feta cheese; 1 ounce baked tofu; 1 small whole grain roll.
Nutrient capsule: High protein, low carbohydrate, low fat,
Food-mood strategy: Enhances mental performance and alertness.

Pick up child at day care center. Plain bagel or flatbread.
Nutrient capsule: High carbohydrate, low protein, low fat.
Food-mood strategy: Alleviates temporary stress quickly.

Dinner. White bean soup; mixed green salad; cornbread; blueberries.
Nutrient capsule: High carbohydrate, low protein, low fat.
Food-mood strategy: Calms after a high-stress day.

Bedtime snack. Whole grain cereal.

Nutrient capsule: High carbohydrate.

Food-mood strategy: Induces relaxation and sleep.[14]

fourteen

Spiritually Imbued Food

When you look at nutrition from a purely scientific
point of view, there is no place for consciousness.
And yet, consciousness could be one of the crucial
determinants of the metabolism of food itself.[1]

—Deepak Chopra, M.D.

As we've seen, for thousands of years mystics, holy people, and
sages have used their consciousness to connect to food's spiritual significance. Now science is beginning to explore what many spiritualists have known intuitively, and religionists have accepted on faith: our
prayers, thoughts—and, perhaps, psychospiritual energy—influence
the food we cultivate, prepare, and eat. In turn, the consciousness we
bring to food may have the potential to become a vital source of
nourishment.

Of Science and Spirituality

Now we have come full circle, to the question provoked by my conversation with Dr. K. L. Chopra: Is it possible to infuse food with spirit? It turns out that, indeed, some researchers have begun to explore the ability of *intentionally directed* thoughts and feelings to transmute energy into our food and, in turn, the possible effects such intentionality may have on both food and our bodies.

I had the opportunity to see this manifest during an unusual dining experience in Europe. At the time, my husband Larry Scherwitz and I were living and working in the ancient, formally Roman town of Neuss, Germany. It was here that we were supervising the lifestyle-change research project based on the work of Dean Ornish, M.D., and colleagues. Larry was the principal investigator on the project; I was the director of nutrition, responsible for training clinical staff in both a rehabilitation clinic in Königsfeld, a small town in northwestern Germany, and in a clinic in southern Holland.

During the preparatory stage of our research, Larry and I met with opinion leaders in Germany's wellness movement at a hotel restaurant in a town north of Düsseldorf, Germany. The purpose: to sample a meal prepared by chefs to whom I had given the program's "no-fat-added," whole foods dietary guidelines. If the meal was tasty, we planned to use the hotel in the future to bring our heart patient group for celebrations.

Participating in the meal were the president and cofounder of the German Wellness Association and his partner; a physician representing AOK, Germany's largest health insurance company; and American physician Leonard Laskow, a colleague from the States who was in Germany to promote his book *Healing with Love*. Trained at New York University School of Medicine and Stanford Medical Center, Dr. Laskow has researched the effects of consciousness on both food and healing.

Before the meal began, Dr. Laskow discussed research he had done with what he refers to as *subtle energy*, the aspect of energy inherent in our bodies, and *holoenergetic* healing, a technique he created that uses this subtle, spiritual energy to heal.

A polite, formal atmosphere had prevailed as Dr. Laskow explained the core belief of his work: that loving energy both outside and inside our bodies could be garnered to enhance the taste of food as well as for healing. That this occurs, he said, could be demonstrated with wine and food. The response at the table was diverse: one health care professional was open and intrigued; another remained distant and observing; yet another was sneeringly skeptical. At Larry's urging, Dr. Laskow offered to demonstrate his technique with the wine sitting on the table before us—an experiment he had replicated hundreds of times during his healing seminars.

The wine in front of us was a red table wine of medium quality, with a distinctly tart aftertaste. To proceed, Larry asked the waiter for two equal-size flasks for the wine, as well as two wine glasses for each guest. Then Dr. Laskow poured similar amounts of the wine into each flask. Next, Larry placed one flask out of range at another table; the second remained in front of Dr. Laskow. Then, with his hands gently surrounding—but not touching—the flask, Dr. Laskow visualized a golden ball of light above his head, then he imagined drawing this "golden" energy through the top of his head into his heart, and transferring the energy from his heart into his hands.

During the next few minutes, he verbally thanked the grapes for "giving of themselves" to be made into wine. He acknowledged the soil for its nourishment, the sun for its energy, and the rain that helped the grapes to grow. Then he acknowledged and thanked the people involved in the grapes-to-wine-to-table process—from the farmer who grew the grapes to the waiter who served it to us.

At this point, Dr. Laskow set the "nourished" flask aside for ten minutes to give it a chance to "restructure." When the ten minutes were up, Larry placed both flasks of wine and the wine glasses on the table, while noting which flask contained the treated wine, and marking the bottom of each wine glass either "treated" or "untreated." Then, after Larry placed a set of "coded" wine glasses before each diner, he poured the "nourished" wine into one set of glasses and the "untreated" wine into the second set.

After each dinner guest had received a "sampling" of both wines, each had their own personal "wine tasting." As with any group process, we went around the table one by one, with everybody paying close attention to everyone else's reaction. One at a time, each person sipped from the two glasses, then commented on any detected differences. Every one of the dinner guests, including myself, was surprised, for had detected and expressed distinct differences in the flavor, body, and aftertaste of the "nourished" vs. "untreated" wine. To me, the nourished wine was smoother, the tart aftertaste gone. It tasted like a better quality, vintage wine.

The wine wasn't the only aspect of the evening that had "reconstructed." As the evening progressed and we drank the wine, we felt the atmosphere at the table change from polite skepticism to a heady euphoria; even the waiter smiled when he approached our table. Although eight of us had shared the one bottle of wine (not enough to be inebriated), there was a palpable feeling of camaraderie and positive energy that had spread among us. Larry, Dr. Laskow, and I believe that the changed atmosphere was due to more than simply the effects of the relatively minor amounts of wine each of us had been served. We think that the energy Dr. Laskow imparted into the wine was also transferred to those who drank it.

This diverse group of academics had experienced and witnessed what appeared to be the channeling of conscious energy into wine. This energy was loving, nonthreatening and peaceful; its essence was spiritual. We had all experienced and witnessed it: Human consciousness or energy (from the *observer*) appeared to have merged with that of the wine (the *observed*), changing its taste—and the mood of the evening, too.

Speculates Dr. Laskow: "If food or wine is infused with love, then when you consume it, or other people ingest it, that change in the structure of the food or liquid could induce similar changes in the structure of the water in your own body. Subjectively, people have told me the taste and fragrance in 'charged' food is different...better. That is also my experience."

Spiritually Imbued Food

Spiritually imbued food is the phrase I use to describe food or liquids that has been transmuted with loving, conscious energy. This can apply to the food on our plates, as well as to all phases of food preparation— from the farmers who grow it, farmhands who harvest it, food manufacturers and transporters, grocers and grocery stores, home cooks and professional chefs, and ultimately us, the diners who reap the nourishment of this collective food consciousness.

As we have seen, the notion that spiritual consciousness (awareness and intention) is integrally connected to food is not a new concept to spiritualists. But to the scientific community, the link between consciousness and food is still in the early stages of exploration. Says author Larry Dossey, M.D., whose books integrate science and spirituality, prayers and healing: "That our consciousness affects matter (including food) is not in doubt. *How* it happens is a huge mystery."[2]

To illuminate our understanding of *how* this may occur, I spoke with Marilyn Schlitz, Ph.D., director of research at the Institute of Noetic Sciences, at her office in Sausalito, California. She describes the Institute as "a think-tank that is dedicated to exploring the interface between science and spirituality"; indeed, the institute defines *noetics* as "consciousness, interiority, and awareness in the broadest sense," and *science* as "empirical investigation based on reproducible evidence." Says Dr. Schlitz: "We make assumptions in the Western world...that plants [and other food] don't have a central nervous system; therefore they're not conscious. But what we do to plants *does* matter," she says emphatically, for human consciousness *does* influence plants and food.

The reason? The interconnectedness of all life. "I think we are all enveloped in an interconnected biosphere," she continues. "And that sound, noise, smells, visuals, light, stimulus...are all relevant to how we're going to be affected. And plants are no different from humans."[3]

Physicist Fred Alan Wolf, Ph.D., concurs. He believes that "we are interconnected in ways that are very subtle and not easy to appreciate." Given this perception, he says that it is insufficient to ask,

"What nutrients are in the food?" Rather, we should also be asking: *"What were you thinking about when you were eating?"*[4] The concept of interconnectedness also asks us to pay attention to that vast concept called *consciousness;* in other words, the thoughts and feelings we bring to food, as well as to everything else in our lives.

Seeking to understand the "how" of the connectedness between our thoughts and various life forms in the last several years, many scientists have conducted a number of well-controlled studies. Some have focused on plants, many of which are edible, while other studies have attempted to assess the effects of thoughts and/or prayer on single-cell organisms such as bacteria and fungus. The core question: Can our thoughts, feelings, and/or consciousness directly influence other living entities, such as soil, plants, and food animals? For if this is so, then it is possible that some form of energy within our own systems can somehow be transferred into our food, changing it from one form into another. The implication is that not only does food affect our bodies, we influence food, too.

What follows is a look into some studies that are giving support to the power of consciousness and its effects on life forms, specifically plants and bacteria. They all imply that a new scientific field is in the making, one that may give us a prescription for creating an as yet unidentified "nutrient" that manifests through the wisdom and awareness we bring to our food.

Plant Talk

Consider the innovative prayer/plant research of Rev. Dr. Karl Goodfellow, minister of the United Methodist Church in Guttenberg, Iowa. What began with children in his church as a "mini-experiment" about the effects of prayer on vegetable seeds evolved into a statewide study in collaboration with researchers at the University of Iowa, his church's congregants, ten thousand intercessors, and his wife Liz, who prayed daily for sixty days for a bountiful harvest and the safety of the one million farmers throughout the state of Iowa.

The idea for such a far-reaching project began on a typical Sunday at Dr. Goodfellow's church when he decided to teach some children how to pray over seeds. To do this, he brought two pans of seeds into the room. "We used pinto beans and Great Northern beans," he explained to me during a phone conversation, "whatever we had in the church pantry." Then they added water to the pans, "hoping to be ready for the springtime," he explained. The children prayed for the seeds before they were planted, while they were still in water. "I asked the children to pray that the seeds would become all that they could become. But we only prayed for half of the germinating seeds; we didn't pray for the other half."

The next step: Dr. Goodfellow planted both the prayed-for and unprayed-for seeds in soil. Placing both sets of plants next to each other, during the next two weeks, "we tried to keep all factors the same: the water, the sunlight, the heat," he said. "Two weeks later the seedlings had grown into small plants," says Liz Goodfellow. "And when we measured them, the unprayed for plants were about two inches tall; the prayed-for plants, about four inches. It was a big difference."

Amazed, they—and others—wondered if the difference was just a fluke. "A science teacher at the local school laughed at our study," says Dr. Goodfellow. "So we ran an experiment there, too. After the children prayed for the seeds in church, they took the prayed-for and unprayed-for seeds over to their school. Again, the prayed-for seeds showed more growth."

Why did the prayed-for seeds grow better? The mechanism is not yet explained scientifically, yet Dr. Goodfellow speculates that some sort of transmission of God's love occurred between the prayers and plants. "When you pray for seeds or a bountiful harvest," he conjectures, "the prayers act as a catalyst. An energy is released that is transmitted to the plants. And the plants, or life forms, respond to that life energy."[5]

"Feeling" Plants

While Dr. Goodfellow explains the transmutation of prayers into the seeds as a release of energy, Cleve Backster, famous for his work showing that plants have "feelings," might describe the prayer/seed experiment as *biocommunication,* one form of intelligent life (humans), communicating with another (plants). Through a fortuitous set of coincidences, Backster revealed that the intention we bring to plants and food affects them. Discussed in *The Secret Life of Plants,* his pioneering work with plants has changed the way many people view plants and food.[6]

A polygraph examiner by trade, Backster had been trained to measure responses of the autonomic nervous system, such as the skin's ability to conduct electricity. Using this and other indirect measures, such as muscle tension and breath, it is possible to draw conclusions about whether a person is lying (in which case, the body is tense), or being truthful (in which case, the body is relaxed). Backster's adventure began one eventful day in the 1960s when he impulsively attached electrodes from his polygraph to the leaf of a *dracaena* plant, a tropical plant with large palm tree-like leaves. After watering the plant, the galvanometer (the part of the lie detector that "writes" the body's response to a question) registered a response.

Amazed, Backster decided to explore the idea that plants may react to how they're treated. Knowing that threatening the well-being of a human is a sure way to cause the polygraph needle to jump, Backster considered making an extreme threat to the leaf that was still attached to the electrodes. His solution: he would dip a leaf from the plant into the hot cup of coffee he held in his hand. But when he did, there was no reaction. Then he perceived a more drastic threat: he would burn the leaf. But he didn't have to. The polygraph needle jumped the moment he merely *imagined* the flame in his mind—even though he had not actually lit the match or moved a muscle. At this point, Backster considered the possibility that plants may be able to differentiate between his *pretending* to cause harm from an authentic *intention* to actually do it.

Intrigued with the idea that plants seemed to have the ability to perceive intention, Backster pursued his polygraph/plant research, which prompted one financial backer of his research to comment that Backster's "work indicates there may be a primary form of instantaneous communication among all living things that transcends physical laws."[7]

Wanting to know more about plant communication, other researchers followed suit, performing hundreds of experiments on plants and food over time. For instance, research chemist Marcel Vogel verified Backster's research when he showed that he could influence plants when he *verbalized* his intention to them; Eldon Byrd, an operations analyst in the United States Navy with a master's degree in medical engineering, studied the cells in leaves, then speculated that human consciousness causes actual changes in plant cells; and Soviet scientists confirmed that the plant-based foods of beans, potatoes, and wheat have "memory," because these foods were able — via pulsations — to repeat the frequency of flashes they received from a xenon-hydrogen lamp.[8] The general consensus: plants seem somehow to sense verbal and nonverbal communication from humans.

Water Wonders

Apparently, water, too, can be affected by focused thoughts and positive intention. Consider the research of Bernard Grad, Ph.D., a research biochemist at a psychiatric institute at McGill University in Montreal. Dr. Laskow, writing in *Healing with Love*, relates that during a series of experiments on plant seedlings, "Dr. Grad had an individual with a 'green thumb' and one severely depressed mental patient each hold a sealed flask of water in their hands." Afterward, Dr. Grad watered some seedlings with the "green thumb"-treated water, some with the water from the depressed patient, and others with plain water that had not been treated. The results: seedlings watered with the "green thumb" water grew fastest; with water from the depressed patient, slowest; those treated with the plain water fell somewhere in between.[9]

As with plants that responded to Backster's thoughts and images, it appears that water also can "store" and "read" information from humans. Given that our bodies are about 66 percent water, the implications of such research are especially profound. If positive and negative thought forms can affect the structure of water *outside* our bodies, they may also impact the billions of cells filled with and surrounded by water *inside* our body.

This research, and similar studies Dr. Grad performed with other psychiatric patients, are relevant for people who plant, grow, harvest, package, or cook food. Dr. Grad theorizes that "if a person's mood could influence a ... solution held in the hands, it seemed natural to assume that a cook's ... mood could influence the quality of food prepared for a meal."[10] Indeed, if a person's emotional state can change water and, in turn, the degree to which a plant thrives, it could also influence the quality of our food—at any stage of its journey to our plate.

Keeping Milk Fresh

It is also possible to use intention and a loving consciousness to influence bacteria in food. During a recent phone conversation, Larry Dossey, M.D., told me that a prayerful, loving intention may also *protect* food from a proliferation of harmful bacteria.[11] Dr. Dossey, the former chief of staff at Humana Medical City Dallas, is the author of pioneering books such as *Prayer is Good Medicine* and *Healing Words,* an overview of the power of prayer (or *intentionality,* as some scientists call it) to heal.

To clarify the concept, he related the story about a group of people from Spindrift, a Florida-based organization that researched prayer and its effects. "They went to Haiti to do ... work with the rural poor, but the people from Spindrift had problems keeping the milk fresh. So they prayed for some sort of refrigeration device to become available. They didn't get the refrigeration device, but after they instituted these prayers, the milk started staying fresh for days longer. So their need was met, but not in the way they thought it would be."

Bacteria's Biocommunication

As the research from Drs. Goodfellow, Backster, Grad, and from Spindrift implies, seeds, seedlings, and food, including milk, seem to be able to respond to our intentions and regard. But what is it about a person's consciousness that seems to influence seedlings, plants, and food? There has been virtually no research on this subject yet; nor is this mystery answered in this book. However, research on the effects of consciousness on simple *non-food* life forms provides some clues about what it is about a cook's consciousness that could affect food.

Scientists have conducted hundreds of quality studies over the years with single-cell organisms, ranging from amoebas and parame-cia to yeast and bacteria. Backster and his colleagues explored the possibility of "cellular communication" by monitoring plants, multi-cellular life forms, with a polygraph and charts. Others, such as Dr. Laskow, researched basic biocommunication with bacteria, a single-cell life form. Described in detail in *Healing with Love,* Laskow's goal was to explore the effects certain intentions, loving energy, and visu-alization could have on tissue culture. Because of the availability of state-of-the-art biochemical techniques—and his interest in healing—he chose tumor cells in culture.

Dr. Laskow shared his research discoveries during a conversation at his home in Mill Valley, California. I was especially interested in speaking with him because when I had once asked him if thoughts affect the molecular structure of food, he had responded, "Of course." Here is a brief overview of his research in his own words:

"I was able to show that by using intention, one can reduce bac-terial growth by 50 percent, compared to controls. I've also shown that I can use loving intention to protect bacteria from the lethal effects of antibiotics. I did this by having the intention to lovingly pro-tect all the bacteria in the solution on which I was focusing. Working in a university laboratory, I had placed bacteria in two sets of test tubes containing an antibiotic. Then I placed the test tubes in the *energy field* that I created between my hands. Basically, my hands were about eight inches apart and the test tubes were between my hands.

"Then I would focus on my heart, while feeling *love* for the bacteria. I would define 'loving energy' as energy that impels us into oneness with the object of our loving awareness; it's coming into a unity with the object of our loving awareness.

"Next, I would lovingly intend to protect all life forms in solution. I would imagine releasing that loving energy and information from my heart and through my hands into the test tubes. I did this by bringing the energy from my heart into my hands with breath. I would take a deep breath, then hold it. And as I released my breath, I would have the intention to transfer the energy and information to the bacteria in the test tube.

"Next I compared the treated bacteria with the control sample, which had the same amount of bacteria, as well as the same amount of antibiotic. The only difference: it had *not* been treated with loving intention. What were the results? The bacteria that I had protected with loving intention was mobile and alive. But the bacteria in the control group were immobile and presumably dead."[12]

Considering the Inconceivable

Intention? Loving the bacteria? Releasing energy? Although such concepts aren't typical components of scientific research, they were major components of Dr. Laskow's studies nonetheless. He discovered that by combining intention, visualization, and loving energy, the bacteria retained vital life energy. Interestingly, when Laskow studied the effects of intention, loving energy, and visualization separately, he found each to have some effect, but they were more potent together.

What may we imply from this research? Is it really feasible for energy to be transferred between two sources—that is, from people to plants and other life forms such as bacteria and rabbits? And if so, what does this imply about the food we eat and the consciousness with which we eat the food?

Says Dr. Laskow: "If you can feel genuine love (unity and connectedness), gratitude, and appreciation before you ingest food, you will be setting the stage for the transformation of that food into every cell in your body. Your spiritual essence is love, and when you have the intention to infuse that love into food, the food is transformed; and that transformed food becomes a part of every cell in your body."

We can speculate that by bringing a prayerful consciousness to food, we're organizing some form of energy in a beneficial, harmonious way. For instance, as we have seen, the plants that received water from the "not depressed" person with a "green thumb" thrived. Apparently, water, plants, and other food may absorb a person's positive prayer properties; in turn, this energy may be given back to us when we eat spiritually imbued food.

Dr. Laskow suggests that when you bring a loving regard to anything, you receive a double dose of the blessing. First you receive the blessing you direct to the food. In turn, this "blessed self" may influence the food or beverage that receives this energy; then when we eat this spiritually imbued food, the loving consciousness imparted to the food may feed the body while, in some special way, also nourishing the soul.

Creating Spiritually Imbued Food

Are these concepts amazing, extraordinary, outrageous, unbelievable? Absolutely—unless you've experienced them for yourself. I had this opportunity when I tasted the difference in Dr. Laskow's "spiritually imbued" wine—as well as in oranges he had treated with loving regard during one of his workshops on consciousness and healing. Projecting loving energy actually changed the taste and texture of the orange—it peeled more readily, and was juicier and sweeter. Dr. Goodfellow and the children in his congregation experienced firsthand the effect that prayers can have on the growth of seedlings. Dr.

Dossey and many other scientists have researched and verified the positive influence a prayerful consciousness can have on single-cell organisms.

Though science is beginning to verify the effects that a loving consciousness—prayers, thoughts, and perhaps, psychospiritual energy—can have on food, it is not necessary to be a scientist to understand and create spiritually imbued food.

What follows are reflections from two people who have performed their own food-related "research"—but not in a laboratory. With the loving consciousness he holds in his heart, Ali Babajane creates spiritually imbued food at his restaurant; *feng shui* practitioner Irene Averell's transcendent link manifests through spiritually infused water, the "elixir" of life that is also a component of virtually all food. Here are their insights in their own words:

Ali Babajane

Born in Iran but raised all over the world, Babajane describes himself as a "food lover." Babajane is the owner of the Champs-Elysées restaurant in Sausalito, California.

"In my heart, I believe that to eat is to make your 'soul sweat.' By this I mean we are activating our connection to the world; we are touching the universe. When I cook, I want to put full love and compassion into it, because this way I am appreciating, and connecting with, the Creator.

"We think we are creating food, but food is actually creating us. I believe that if you cook food with love, compassion, and awareness, this consciousness goes through your hands—while you're cutting the vegetables, the meat. It's transferable. If you think about it, everything on this planet has energy that can never be destroyed. It will only be transferred to something else, such as food. Definitely.

"I've seen this with my own eyes. Every time I cook food, if I'm angry or negative, no matter how many herbs or spices I put in...and the aroma is nice...the table is silent. They eat the food, but the people are silent. The food does not have the glory...the *oomph!* And so the people eating it don't respond. They don't talk much. Something is flat.

"But when I go into my kitchen and prepare the food with loving awareness, when I have a party or friends come over, they're rowdy and laughing. They'll eat whatever I serve and enjoy it. They just go crazy with a joyous spirit.

"This happens because everything is connected. So any time we eat, it gives us energy to walk, talk, think. And when you eat food imbued with either negative or positive loving thoughts, that same energy is transferred from our minds, hearts, and souls into our food. Then once the food is in our bodies, this energy is transferred back again into our minds, hearts, and souls.

"Most of us have our own ritual and recipes when we prepare food. The only difference is the energy we transfer throughout the food. When this energy is loving, the food will digest well in the body. This is because the mind, soul, and heart have picked up the loving energy in the food. The opposite happens, though, if the food is prepared with negativity. It will be tasteless and harder to digest.

"When I visited Mazandaran, a province in northern Iran, I watched people who were growing onions. On a day when the farmer was angry, I put a stick right in the soil next to the onions he planted that day. And the next day, when he was smiling and giggling, I put another stick next to the onions he planted that day, too. Afterward, I tasted them. One was hard and tasteless; the other sweet and tasty. They had both been grown in the same soil, with the same water. Yet they were different.

"Food is similar to art. When you look at a good painting, first you see the color. Second, you look at the composition. Next, you ask yourself, What is the message in the painting? With food, the first thing that reaches us is the aroma. The second is the color. The third is taste. When you taste the food, then you know the consciousness with which it was prepared. Then you know the magnitude of it, the meaning of the food. This is what goes through your body and sticks to your soul.

"I believe we should cook with the consciousness that we are feeding the world. Because this is what we're doing each time we prepare food. When you feed others, you are feeding yourself. Because everything you give is given back to you. So through food, you are creating the most incredible positive magnet that makes us all one. This is why we should all use love as an ingredient in the food we prepare and eat. Not only is it a gift to others, it's a gift to ourselves, too."[13]

Irene Averell

Feng shui is an ancient Chinese art dealing with the energy flow in your environment (home, office, etc.), and its effects on your life. While attending a retreat, Irene learned to create what she refers to as "wholy" water.

"To help clients manifest their dreams and create miracles in their lives, I attended a five-day retreat to learn how to tap into unseen energies. At one of the workshops, twenty of us stood in a circle as our teacher poured water from a pitcher into the two small cups each of us was holding. We set one cup aside; the other, we continued to hold in our hands. Then we were told to project all the love we could muster into the water-filled cup in our hands. To conjure up loving feelings, some of us thought of special people in our lives; others focused on pets; still others filled their hearts with God.

"Then each of us poured the 'love-treated' water into the original pitcher. When the pitcher was full, the teacher repoured the collective love-treated water back into our cups. Next, we were asked to pick up the cup of water we had set aside and taste it; then to drink the love-treated water.

"The tastes were entirely different. The 'untreated' water tasted like standard tap water. But the 'treated' water...well...it had been blessed. People said it went down their throats like silk. It was sweet. Some said they felt euphoric at the thought of having drunk this blessed water. Others felt their eyes well up with tears, because they were so profoundly touched by the thought that loving energy could be shared through water, one of life's vital 'elixirs.'

"Now in my *feng shui* work, I use *wholy* water when I bless homes or work spaces. By infusing water with the light of love, I replace any negative energy there may be. Whatever the desired outcome—perfect health, prosperity, a sense of harmony—you can transfer the positive outcome you want into the water—and then drink it.

"Since returning home, I often reflect on the effect our collective loving energy had on the water—how it had changed the water's taste; what it felt like to drink it. I recall the sensation of the blessed *wholy* water going from my lips, into my mouth, down my throat and 'into my heart.' And then I think about how it felt as it 'spread' through my body, then throughout the room and out into the universe."[14]

Self-Test Strategies

Consider creating your own spiritually imbued food. While holding awareness of the food and a loving intention in mind, try some of these "mini-experiments" and see if you can detect a difference in the spiritually imbued food you create in your own kitchen.

- *Processed vs. hand-prepared veggies.* Make a multicolored salad with some of your favorite vegetables, perhaps carrots, mushrooms, tomatoes, cucumbers, celery, and some dark leafy greens. Chop half of the vegetables by hand, using a knife and cutting board; cut up the other half in a food processor. Can you detect a difference in taste between the vegetables that were touched with loving regard, compared with those processed in the food processor?

- *Cooking consciously vs. unconsciously.* Before enjoying a favorite dish, shop for, prepare, cook, and eat the food with a loving consciousness. As a contrast, the next time you prepare the same dish, choose to do so during an especially busy time in your life. For instance, perhaps it's a weekday when you didn't carve out enough time to purchase, prepare, and eat the food. In addition, the loving regard was missing. Can you detect any difference between the "regarded" and "unregarded" dishes? Do they taste different? Also, how did you feel—both physically and psychologically—after consuming each dish?

- *"Treated" vs. "untreated" beverages.* Review Dr. Laskow's wine experiment and "method" that follow. Then repeat it with any beverage of choice, such as water, juice, or wine. After the "treated" beverage has had some time to "restructure"—perhaps ten minutes—see if you can taste any differences between the "treated" and "untreated" beverage.

Laskow's Method

Here in more detail and in his own words, is Leonard Laskow's method of infusing liquids and food with loving energy.

Intentionality. "To become present, bring your attention to your breath. Be aware of when you're breathing in and breathing out. By becoming aware of your breathing, you can take voluntary control over a largely involuntary process. And as you become aware of your breathing—letting your breath occupy your mind—you're holding and then releasing the *intention* to relax. And then your body begins to relax."

Heart focus. "Focus your attention on your heart center, imagining that you are breathing in and out through your chest. To further enhance the meditative state, engage the energy of your heart center by conjuring up deep, loving, caring feelings. To conjure up such feelings, you may want to recall a loving experience. For instance, you may have felt a sense of loving unity during a walk in nature, when you were with a special person, or while listening to a profoundly moving piece of music."

Letting in the light. "To enhance the sense of loving energy emanating from the heart, envision a shimmering sphere of light—similar to the sun—several inches above your head. Imagine the energy from this glistening light entering through the crown of your head, cascading down to your heart and hands, then overflowing out through your heart and hands. This visualization is designed to help you transcend your identification with your body, and realize that you're more than your body, feelings, or thoughts."

Food infusion. "Once this loving energy and 'light' is flowing through you, have the *intention* of projecting it onto the food [or beverage]. Visualize this is happening. Have the intention that the loving energy and light is coming out through your heart and infusing the food—like a searchlight that is shining on the food. You can also surround both sides of the dish [or glass] with your hands, and imagine energy coming from both hands into the food [or beverage]."[15]

fifteen

Food Meditation: Creating Conscious Connection

To receive the most subtle particles in the food, you must be fully conscious, wide awake, full of love. If the entire system is ready to receive food in that perfect way, then the food is moved to pour out its hidden riches...when food opens itself, it gives you all that it has in the way of pure, divine energies.[1]

—O. M. Aivanhov

I was looking at the fruit in the basket and I started to feel the fruit kind of giving itself up to the world.... I could feel the essence of the fruit. I swear to you, I could. And I had to stop myself from crying from looking at the fruit.... I was so grateful for the little pomegranates and their seeds.[2]

—Oprah Winfrey

When you're not paying attention—are not "fully conscious"—food is merely something to eat. But blend the produce on your plate with the food-related, meditative wisdom of various traditions, cultures, and science—and both you and the food you consume may be transformed. In place of mundane munching, the act of eating becomes "sense-filled," then may go beyond what the senses can perceive to what in mysticism is called **non-sense**[3]—that which the ordinary senses cannot perceive. What follows are two food meditation methods: one from Buddhist tradition; another with Taoist roots. They are designed to further enhance your ability to create your own personal conscious connection to food.

Eating Meditation

In the gentle light of the meditation room, forty patients, all referred by their doctors, are sitting in a circle studying the two raisins each holds in the palm of one hand. Jon Kabat-Zinn, Ph.D., the class' instructor, has just distributed the raisins with a spoon from a hand-carved bowl made for him twenty-five years ago by a friend (now a pediatrician at Yale University) from his days in graduate school, when he studied molecular biology at the Massachusetts Institute of Technology.

On a stormy day, at a cafe in San Francisco, I spoke with Dr. Kabat-Zinn about the mindfulness meditation model he created, designed to show people how to become more fully awake and perceive the vividness of each moment.[4] A meditator himself since 1966, he uses his particular approach at his Stress Reduction Clinic at the University of Massachusetts Medical Center, now part of the newly created Center for Mindfulness and Medicine, Health Care and Society. Written about in his books *Full Catastrophe Living* and *Wherever You Go, There You Are,* Kabat-Zinn's mindfulness and stress reduction program is now in use in more than a hundred hospitals and clinics around the country, as well as by sports teams and even some prisons.

To give each person embarking on this journey of self-discovery an experiential, hands-on sense of what it means to meditate mindfully, Dr. Kabat-Zinn often starts off through an exploration of the senses, using an ordinary experience such as eating. This "eating meditation" serves to dispel any mystical or romantic ideas people may have about meditation, while at the same time revealing its power and potential through its ordinariness. Here is one mindfulness meditation (originally learned from Buddhist teacher Jack Kornfield) in Kabat-Zinn's own words:

Sight. "To begin, I ask the people in the class, who are almost all new to meditation, to look at the raisin while imagining they are Martian scientists who just parachuted down to Earth and had never seen one before. To look at it carefully without naming it. Sometimes — following Buddhist teacher Thich Nhat Hanh — I'll ask if they can see the water, the rain, and the sunlight within each raisin. Or the earth. When they're ready, they'll tell me what they're seeing. For instance, some describe the raisin as 'wrinkly' or 'brown.'"

Smell. "Next I'll ask them to bring the raisin up to their noses. Some may say the scent is 'musky'; others describe it as 'sweet.' What's important is the experience itself, not the word that describes the scent."

Physiological reaction. "Now we focus on what's going on in their mouths. People begin to notice that salivation is happening — even though they haven't put the raisin in their mouths yet. They're noticing a mind/body phenomenon — the senses responding just to the *anticipation* that something's going to be eaten. That alone causes our glands to secrete saliva."

Touch. "Now we explore how the raisins feel. Some describe them as 'soft'; others say they're 'squishy.'"

Motion and movement. "We also notice the *proprioceptive* sense (sensing the body in space) of where the body is. How is it that the hand actually knows how to get the raisin to the lips, without going past the face altogether? Although the cerebellum controls gross motor activity, it's completely unconscious. Unless we are paying close attention, we take it for granted that our hand knows how to deliver the raisin to our lips.

"As we bring the raisin up to the lips, we notice what happens next. As with the proprioceptive sense, the mouth receives the raisin. Nothing goes into the mouth without its being received. And who or what is doing the receiving? The tongue.

"Now watch what the tongue is doing with it. How does it get the raisin between the teeth? It's amazing that the tongue is so skilled, such a remarkable muscle that it can actually receive food and then keep it between the teeth. The cheek working on one side, the tongue working on the other. This all happens totally below the level of consciousness."

Taste. "After becoming aware of the raisin in our mouth, we actually start biting into it…slowly. Then we begin to chew. Some will notice that the tongue decides which side of the mouth it's going to chew on. Putting all our attention in our mouth, we take a few bites. Then we stop to experience what's happening. And what's happening is invariably an *explosion* of taste.

"I ask people to express what's going on. To be really refined. What is the experience? Some say 'sweet,' or 'sour,' or 'juicy.' There are hundreds of words that describe this experience we call 'tasting.'"

Texture. "As they continue to chew, the taste changes. And so does the consistency. At a certain point, they become aware of the texture of the raisin. Because the taste is kind of gone. The texture becomes …a bit aversive actually, and you may want to swallow it."

Swallowing. "But we don't have people swallow it yet. We ask them to stay with the aversion—as well as the impatience and the inborn impulse to swallow. We ask them not to swallow until they detect the impulse to do so. And then to observe what is involved in actually getting the food over to the place where it's going to be swallowed.

"When they detect the impulse to swallow, I say, 'And now, in your mind's eye, follow it down into the stomach, and feel your whole body, and acknowledge one way or another that your body is now exactly one raisin heavier.' And they do this."

Breath. "Next, after a pause for a moment or two, we ask them to see if they can 'taste' their breath in a similar way, to bring the same quality of attention they gave to seeing the raisin, feeling the raisin, smelling the raisin, tasting the raisin.... Now bring that to the breath.

"And from here, then we drop into silence. By this point, people understand something of what meditation is. It's doing what we do all the time, except we're doing it with attention. Directed, moment-to-moment, nonjudgmental attention.

"By now, ten minutes or more have passed. And the group is about to begin the same mindfulness meditation process again with the second raisin that is still being held in their hand."

Ancient/New Meditation

Meditation. In the East, yogis say it leads to a superconscious state that emerges from the cessation of thought; Taoists tell us it is "to come into harmony with all things and all moments,"[5] that it is the way to return to the depths within the self; while believers of Zen present it as a path to sudden illumination.[6] In the West, it has more often been linked to the mystical and monastical. The *Cabala*, a Jewish mystical teaching, turns to it to carry consciousness through various "gateways"; early Christian monks and saints used it as a stringent contemplative process to achieve spiritual exaltation; and Islam's mystical Sufis interpret it repetitiously, to suffuse their mind, heart, and soul with "higher things."[7]

This ancient tradition comes from the Latin *meditari*, which implies "deep, continued reflection, a concentrated dwelling in thought."[8] But while it is often linked with the concept of contemplation, the meditative process may also involve emptying the mind (*apophatic* meditation) by eliminating thoughts from consciousness. Still another form of meditative practice (*cataphatic*) entails holding a specific image, idea, or word in the "mind's eye," allowing emotions to center in the heart.[9]

There are many roads that lead to the serenity at the summit of the "meditation mountain." The mindfulness meditation practiced by Dr. Kabat-Zinn finds its roots in the Buddhist tradition. Believed to promote a sense of tranquility and refined awareness (as do all meditation methods), the practice of mindfulness is experienced through four areas: the body, sensation, thought, and objects (such as raisins and other food).

For instance, during the "raisin meditation," focusing on the breath, which came at the end of the process, brought attention to the *body*, as did considering the motion involved in placing the raisin—the *object*—into the mouth; attention on *sensations* was evident through awareness of the raisin in the mouth, chewing, and the urge to swallow it; and mindfulness of *thought* manifested through people in the group expressing their opinions and reactions to various stages of the "raisin meditation."

Whether the source of meditation techniques comes from ancient Eastern or Western traditions—or the modern trend to merge meditation techniques with medicine to manage stress—the goal is the same: to enhance relaxation and self-awareness, and suffuse the mind, heart, and soul with a sense of unity and union with the Absolute.

Says Dr. Kabat-Zinn: "Meditation is actually a process of nourishment, an oxygen line straight into the soul. It is the universe expressing through you, making it an aspect of the sacred."

Eating from a Place of Spirit

In the West, we may describe the energy that manifests this spiritual transformation as a release of endorphins, chemical "messengers" released in the brain that make us feel relaxed, connected, "unanxious." In China, though, the concept of *chi* (the life-force within all living things, from feelings to food) is used to describe what clinical psychologist Michael Mayer, Ph.D., calls "the universal mother," that "energy potential in the world that is soothing, giving us a sense of merging with" the mysterious energy source that is life itself.[10] Indeed, the cultivation of *chi* is both an art and science, capable of unleashing insights, intuition, and a sense of unity—between mind and body, self, and world.

Dr. Mayer, director of the Psychotherapy and Healing Center in Berkeley, California, has been practicing Taoist meditation since 1974. In addition to his clinical practice, he is dedicated to what he describes as "bringing ancient sacred wisdom traditions into modern life." He is also a teacher of T'ai Chi and Chi Kung, ancient forms of moving meditation used in China for centuries to create mind/body balance. After attending one of his T'ai Chi classes, I knew he would have much to offer about meditation, *chi*, and their connection to food in our lives. As we talked on the phone from our respective offices, he shared his penetrating insights.

Consider Dr. Mayer's explanation about how *chi* is based on *how* and *when* we eat: "Eating has both soul and spirit," he told me. For instance, "when we eat something that tastes really good, it touches our soul...helping us to connect to our own humanity, to the earth itself, and its gifts. We become aware of the pleasure of the senses, our taste awakens, we relish the fullness of imbibing life.

"Or, consider how we feel when we eat lightly...we don't get as much of a 'crash down' after eating [as we would with heavier foods]. Instead, we start to feel our spirit rise. If you meditate before eating, then you're eating with awareness and serenity, from a place of spirit."

What does it mean to "eat from that place of spirit?" It would mean being "present with your eating," says Dr. Mayer, "and not taking the food for granted. Every single taste in the food would be more appreciated. And when we appreciate something, our hearts are open. And when our hearts are open, perhaps the food would taste better. *Perhaps the chemistry in our body would metabolize the food differently"* [emphasis added].

"Heartfelt" Eating

To eat with such heartfelt energy—or *chi*—is one of the major intentions of meditation. "When we meditate," explains Dr. Mayer, "distinctions dissolve...and we return to our own true nature. We enter into a state that is blissful...and start to feel a oneness with all that is around. We feel connected to ourselves, others, and the universe itself. Taoist masters refer to this opening up as *energy gates,*" which is a metaphor for entering a more aware, conscious state. Such a change is "alchemical," he continues, "in that the self transforms into something more vital."

To eat—or do anything, for that matter—with such vitality and awareness is to eat with what Dr. Mayer says is "a strong felt-sense." This means that by meditating, you have "activated your personal *chi* in such a way that it merges with the larger *chi* of the universe."

Charging the Chi

To activate *chi* and approach food "from that place of spirit," Dr. Mayer teaches a Taoist meditation technique called *Yichuan.* Developed by Wang Xian Zhai, it is a system of Chi Kung, designed to concentrate the spirit and stabilize the mind through a series of standing postures and movements.[11]

Basically, Yichuan is a simple—but potent—meditation practice that leads to focusing intention on the process of eating: taking the time to be present in the moment, being conscious of an inner illumination that is based on an awareness of the spiritual depths within and without, and an appreciation of the food. Says Dr. Mayer, "When I do this, it feels as if I'm praying over my food. I can actually feel the energy in the room transform."

Dr. Mayer continues: "When I'm dining with my family, I may say a prayer. But I might say a different kind of prayer if I'm eating by myself. If I'm with other people, while I'm talking and enjoying the company, I'll 'drop in' by consciously appreciating the food that I'm eating. Or I might pause, taste the food, and consider if I'm still hungry or 'just right.'

"Each dining experience has its own *intention.* What's important is to remain aware, on some level, of the food and how you're feeling." And how you're breathing. For when you're aware of the cycle of breathing in and breathing out, "something flowers inside," says Dr. Mayer. "Your *chi* is released and you feel the 'bloom' of inner peace...and sense of oneness."

To create your own Yichuan food meditation, Dr. Mayer suggests the following, derived from an ancient Taoist technique:

Balance your breath with this breathing technique:

- Begin by breathing gently, rhythmically, and slowly.

- Continuing to breath gently, place your tongue lightly against the palate, resting the tip just behind the top teeth.

- As you breath in, imagine the breath (energy) traveling up your spine, to your head, and then going over the top of your head.

- As you exhale, imagine the breath going down the front of your body, until it comes down to the perineum, the lowest point in the center of the pelvic area.

- After exhaling, pause briefly before inhaling again.

- Develop a "long breath" while inhaling and exhaling.

(Note: Long breaths, rather than short and choppy breathing, are what activate the *chi.* You will *not* experience *chi* if your breathing is shallow.)

- Position your hands as if there were a small beach ball on top of your food, and your hands are holding that beach ball.

- Keeping your hands in this position, let go of your thoughts about the day. Let go of stress. Let go of wanting to rush to eat before the food gets cold—or any other distractions.

Activate attention

- Focus on the food, appreciating the beautiful designs created by the different colors in the food—the orange of the carrots, the red of the tomatoes—and the process that brought it from the earth to you.

- As you are relaxing and letting go of thoughts, an altered state (a change from a normal state of consciousness) emerges. Be open to experiencing the energy in your own body, and how it feels to have it merge with the energy of the universe.

- As you open up your own appreciation, your heart opens. And as your heart opens, you enter an altered state, a transcendent state, filled with a sense of appreciation and love for the food.

- With your hands still "rounded," and continuing with long, rhythmic breaths, focus your attention and awareness on the food. Continue to feel an appreciation for the food.

- If you're dining with others, give your attention to the circle of togetherness. Consider that the food is a focal point for camaraderie, for connecting with others.

- If alone, appreciate the food and its ability to nourish you.

Reflections on Food

"In farming, as in gardening...if you treat the land with love and respect...it will repay you in kind," says England's Prince Charles, referring to the philosophy behind his line of organic, herbal sparkling waters.[12] He is not alone in his belief that food and humankind share a symbiotic connection. For as we have seen throughout this book, a plethora of cultures, religionists, spiritualists and scientists also create conscious connections to food, and share a reverence for food and the spiritual rewards it can reap.

But it is not necessary to define yourself through a specific religion or culture to achieve a sense of connectedness through food. Nor is it necessary to formally meditate. Many pursue a spiritual relationship to food through what author Sue Bender calls the "everyday sacred."[13] Whether growing, harvesting, cooking, serving, or consuming food, it is possible to instinctively and intuitively relate to food with loving regard. In turn, as consciousness permeates the food, it lends its spirit back to you. In this way, food nourishes both body and spirit—and vice versa—and the cycle of life continues.

For Valerie Phipps, such a spiritual relationship to food manifests through the food she grows and harvests on her farm. With her husband Tom and partner Margarito Ortega, Valerie owns a fifty-acre organic farm in Pescadero, California, a small town located about an hour south of San Francisco. Here, in her own words, are her food-related reflections. May her insights serve as a reflection into your own soul, a guidepost for creating your own spiritual ingredients.

"We started farming in 1969, but we've been growing heritage beans since 1980. Today we grow more than forty-five varieties. Heritage beans are also called heirloom beans. Some varieties were brought to America by people who immigrated here; others were native to North America and part of the Native American Indian heritage. Some beans, such as lentils and soy, may go back thousands of years.

"Not too long ago, the Anasazi bean was found stored in ancient cliff dwellings in Colorado. Since 130 AD, the Anasazi Indians lived in the Four Corners area of Colorado, Arizona, Utah, and New Mexico. Even though the beans had been stored for hundreds of years, they were still able to grow. Perhaps this is because they were in a dry, arid environment. There was no moisture to attack the germ, so it stayed alive.

"Our beans come from as far away as Africa and Central America; about seven or eight varieties were cultivated by Natives. When the white settlers came to America...the Natives would give them beans to survive. The winters were hard, and until the settlers learned the land, Native Americans would provide them with food, including beans.

"At our farm, we have a large area that we set aside for children. We let them sit down in a large pile of beans, then we teach them how to shell the beans. They're so excited because they always thought beans came from cans. We talk a lot about what farmers really do.

"A true farmer loves the land. When you till the soil, you have a connection to the land and the elements: water, sun, air, earth, all working together to help grow the crop that you are going to provide to the world.

"The beans we grow here on Phipps Ranch are planted by hand. They are cultivated by hand and then are harvested, cleaned, and sorted by hand. By the time they are ready to be sold, they have been touched by the hands of many people.

"I believe that the energy of the humans who touched those beans goes into the beans as well. They become vibrant because of the handling. This vibrancy is something that a machine or harvester doesn't have. From my standpoint...I believe that if food is grown and prepared with love...infused with love...well, it can be the humblest of foods, but because it's prepared with love, it's special.

"Food prepared with love is very different from food that's prepared by someone who doesn't care, or because it's a job. Then it's just a meal and you slam it on the table, expecting people to eat it. I don't think that people who eat this food would get nearly as much out of it as those who eat a meal that was prepared with love and respect for all the ingredients that went into the preparation and cooking of that food.

"An old farm magazine tells the story of an old grandmother who prepared the meals on a farm. Just before the food was ready to be cooked or baked, Grandma would take a container out of the cupboard, open the lid, and put a pinch of what was in the container into every dish she made. When she died, her family went through the cupboard. And when they found the container, they looked inside. It was empty—except for the word *love* which they found on a lone piece of paper.

"I believe in this story—that putting love into food makes a difference. Because over the years, I've had so much feedback from people who tell us our beans are wonderful. They tell us our beans are beautiful, that there are no other beans like them."[14]

Creating Conscious Connection

Each time we approach food—whether in gardening, shopping, cooking, or eating—we are presented with an opportunity to visit the meditative consciousness and make the experience "an aspect of the sacred." Throughout this book, there has been a plethora of suggestions designed to enhance this connection. As a last guide, we may turn to the meditative methods described here, or a potpourri of other time-honored meditative methods. Or we may choose to create our own unique approach for making a conscious connection to food.

Adopting meditation's theoretical accessories, by themselves, isn't the goal; rather, such methods serve as the vehicle upon which our spirits can soar, so we may receive the physical, psychological, and spiritual nourishment inherent in all of our food-related activities.

Keep in mind that the process entails regarding food and its preparation as sacred, and bringing an appreciative awareness and sense of sincerity to food. To cultivate such a regard, take the time to be focused and present in the moment while, at the same time, feeling a sense of gratitude for all the people and the processes involved in bringing the food to your kitchen. Also regard, honor, and appreciate the role of nature itself: the sun, rain, and soil that nurtured the food.

Another aspect of bringing a loving regard to food is in how you handle it. Bring a loving awareness to each step of the preparation, from shopping to serving to eating and the after-meal clean-up. Do your best not to allow any distractions to divert your focus, attention, and intention. As important, do not be time-urgent when you practice bringing a prayerful consciousness to food. When you're rushing, your thoughts are elsewhere. And if you're not "in the moment," the food will not receive the appropriate energy. Remember: intention, love or gratitude, and awareness are key concepts for imbuing food with spiritual energy.

Minding the Mystery

Exploring our spiritual connectedness to food is a lifetime adventure, one we may take each time we grow, harvest, handle, cook, or eat food. When we bring a loving awareness to our meals, food holds the potential to nurture within us a soul-satisfying connection to something larger than ourselves. Indeed, it serves to remind us that food is a "medium" between nature and ourselves, and that imbuing food with feelings and intentional thought implies an interrelationship among ourselves and other living entities—soil, plants, food animals, food "intermediaries" such as farmers, truckers, grocers, and chefs, and friends and families.

As we experience this connection, along with absorbing food's nutrients comes the possibility of integrating the consciousness of all who have had contact with the food—including our own. In this way, the food we eat may help us to stumble across our—and life's—true essence: the unity and oneness of all life suggested by saints, mystics, and scientists alike.

Enlightened Eating

I have found that many who practice the principles of enlightened eating are already on the path toward creating a strong spiritual relationship to food. They select fresh, whole, "live" food (fruits, vegetables, whole grains, legumes, nuts, and seeds) as often as possible. They also tend to eat consciously, retaining an awareness and appreciation of the relationship between their bodies and food. They savor their food before eating by regarding and appreciating it. And they chew slowly. They also create a peaceful, calm environment while dining, which often includes agreeable conversation among friends or family members. If alone, they eat in silence, without the distraction of reading material or television. They respect their bodies, eating only when hungry and unrushed; they stop eating when they begin to feel full. And after a meal, they often spend a bit of time savoring the sense of nourishment and "afterglow."

Jon Kabat-Zinn reminds us that "if you look deeply into one thing, you can see everything else. If you look at a raisin or an orange, you can see the sunlight...rain, earth, the farmer, the vine, or the tree the food grew on, the people who pick, pack, and truck it. Every one of those elements has to be part of the food in order for it to come into your hands and then into your body.... So if you go into a store and simply buy an orange, you have an opportunity to realize that you are completely imbedded into a network, a web, an opportunity to realize how deeply interconnected we all are."

Psychologist Michael Mayer says that "when you meditate before eating, you're eating from that place of spirit and appreciation. And when you appreciate something, your heart is open, and the chemistry of the body, I imagine, burns food in a different way. Experimentally, it's like a higher octane gas that burns with less residue."

Dr. Leonard Laskow says that "if we meditate lovingly on food, and we have a sense of deep, honest appreciation for it...and we eat that food, that food, in turn, nourishes us with love...to the extent that our consciousness allows it."

Interconnectedness. Spirit and body chemistry. Loving intention. Living with an awareness of oneness with all aspects of life — including each other and food—lies at the heart of enlightened eating and the mystery of food's ability to nourish both body and soul. By approaching food meditatively and with loving intention, we may go beyond the level of thought and intuit the sacred connection between Mother Earth, food, and humankind. In this way, all of the traditions and methods in this book help us to perceive food as a life force, a nurturer, a gift that recharges and sustains...if we take the time to listen to the message that emerges from the union of food, body, and soul.

acknowledgments

To reveal meanings that underlie food-related beliefs and rituals, I interviewed more than forty-five people who shared their expertise, insights, and time. I am grateful to all of them for contributing to the creation of this book.

Rabbi Harold Schulweis of Valley Beth Shalom synagogue in Encino, California, "demystified" Jewish dietary wisdom by offering insights into Judaism's regard and compassion for all life, especially that of food animals. Richard Schwartz, Ph.D., stayed in close touch with me during the writing of the book, keeping me posted about his vegetarian-based advocacy work with the Jewish community in both the United States and Israel, and also contributed an invaluable critique of the chapter. Roberta Kalechofsky, Ph.D., expanded my awareness about Jewish values and their relationship to animal rights.

Father Robert Bryant of the Episcopal Church of Our Saviour in Mill Valley, California, offered creative insights about the spiritual essence behind the taking of the Eucharist. Professor and theologian Clayton Harrop, Ph.D., contributed historical and symbolic perspectives on the meaning of meals, bread, and wine for early Christians. Former Franciscan monastic Jean Molesky-Poz communicated much care and compassion about her personal beliefs that surround the taking of the bread and wine of the Eucharist. My friend Arthur Manetta, Jr. helped me understand the profound meaning and "real life" relevance inherent in the liturgy of the Eucharist. Jerry and JoAnna Scherwitz, my in-laws, have my deepest respect and appreciation for sharing a "Eucharist consciousness" with family and friends, and those beyond their community. I also thank Doug Campbell, a theology student at Golden Gate Seminary in Mill Valley, California, for his library support.

Restaurateur Adolf Dulan and homemaker Mrs. Clementine Bradshaw welcomed me into their "soul food kitchens." They taught me how to infuse food with love and in the process enhance food's textures, color, scent, and taste—and the enjoyment of it with family and friends.

Hindu physician K. L. Chopra, M.D., Swami Dharmananda, and yoga practitioner Nischala Joy Devi discussed the spiritual beliefs that underlie the "science" of yogic nutrition. I thank them for their shared wisdom and their insights into this ancient tradition.

I am grateful to Ahmad Sakr, Ph.D., nutritionist, author, and founder of the Foundation for Islamic Knowledge, for his heartfelt help. When I contacted Dr. Sakr to request an interview for this book, he made an extraordinary gesture: he asked me to send him a copy of my questions. After receiving them, he took the time to give detailed answers to all of my questions on an audiocassette recording that he kindly sent to me. Dr. Sakr also carefully reviewed the chapter, offered supplemental information, and sent me literature about food and Islam along with two of his books. Mrs. Ameena Jandali welcomed me into her home, shared much with me about her own and her family's food-related Muslim practices, and patiently reviewed the chapter with me to ensure accuracy. Hamid Algar, Ph.D., a professor at the University of California, Berkeley, educated me about the food beliefs of Islam's mystical Sufis.

With Tibetan High Lama Rinpoche, I traveled—in spirit—to Tibet before much of its culture was destroyed by China. He taught me about the spiritual essence of the "butter sculptures" that are unique to Tibetan monastics. Tibetan nun Carol Corradi helped me to appreciate food-related Tibetan Buddhist beliefs. Zen Buddhist Yvonne Rand explained much about both Tibetan and Zen Buddhist food philosophies. Konrad Ryushin Marchaj of the Zen Mountain Monastery and Dharma Communications took the time to edit the section about the *Oryoki* monastic meal to ensure its accuracy.

Writer Suk Wah Bernstein introduced me to the magic of the Chinese New Year's "midnight meal." Christie Bartlett and Scott McDougall of the Urasenke Foundation taught me the subtle delights inherent in the Way of Tea (called the Japanese tea ceremony by

Westerners). Emiko Sekino, her mother, and grandmother, of the Soko Nichibeikai tea house in San Francisco, graciously explained the intricacies and tradition of the Way of Tea. David Lee Hoffman, proprietor of Silk Road Teas, infused my senses with an appreciation of the history and subtleties of Chinese tea.

By sharing her memorable, personal experience of fasting while on a vision quest, Native American Katie Martin showed me how abstaining from food can teach us how to step back from always having to *do* in order to just *be* in the world of the Great Spirit.

Yoga teacher Nutan Brownstein, who is from Bombay, India, told me about her extraordinary Hindu wedding feast—and the "feast within the feast" that occurs while nuptials are exchanged. She and her husband Arthur patiently reviewed the chapter and added relevant details about the fabulous food at both their feast and their marriage altar. Pandit Dabral of the Himalayan Institute added to my understanding of the centuries-old symbolism and spiritual significance that surrounds food at the Hindu wedding.

I also am grateful to the specialists who talked with me about what I call *psychological nutrition,* including food-mood research and the study of eating disorders. I originally talked with food-mood expert Catherine Christie, Ph.D., R.D., (of Nutrition Associates) when I interviewed her for a magazine article I wrote about the effects of food on mood; Dr. Christie graciously agreed to let me include her insights in this book. Psychologist Susan Boulware, Ph.D., who specializes in eating disorders, shared her expertise and reviewed the chapter for accuracy.

I feel privileged and grateful to have had the opportunity to learn about and discuss the spiritual elements of food and nutrition research from specialists in the field, pioneers in their exploration about the mystery of consciousness and food—and the divine life that is inherent in both. Author Larry Dossey, M.D., who has done much research and writing about prayer and consciousness, talked with me about the effect of consciousness and prayers on food. He referred me to Rev. Dr. Karl Goodfellow of the United Methodist Church. Rev.

Goodfellow is collaborating with the University of Iowa on a research project that studies the influence of prayer on food, and he shared their unique work with me. Marilyn Schlitz, Ph.D., director of research at the Institute of Noetic Sciences, contributed her unique experience and perspective about consciousness and food.

I am indebted to Leonard Laskow, M.D., who shared his knowledge about consciousness and food, and the techniques he developed that are designed to help us "connect" with food; psychologist and T'ai Chi practitioner Michael Mayer, Ph.D., who provided insights about the ancient concept of *chi* energy and food; and Jon Kabat-Zinn, Ph.D., author and stress management expert, who taught me about Zen meditation and its application to food. Drs. Laskow, Mayer, and Kabat-Zinn also shared their unique food-related meditation techniques.

It is with pleasure, too, that I thank (heritage bean) farmer Valerie Phipps, restauranteur Ali Babajane, and *feng shui* specialist Irene Averell for sharing their profound insights and experiences with me about the spiritual significance of food in their lives. By stopping their own internal dialogue, they have been able to hear (and share) wisdom about the "creation," the life, that is in food.

Stephen Sparler, who is knowledgeable about religion, science, and spirituality, shared his expertise and opinions; he also edited certain chapters in the book and, as always, offered erudite insights. Deanna Quinones, too, offered invaluable editorial support.

I also want to express appreciation and regard for the support and help given to me by my friend Amy Gage. She encouraged me throughout, always finding time in her busy schedule to put me in touch with appropriate people and books. Also invaluable was the ongoing encouragement and enthusiasm given to me by my friend Linda Gibbs, who is also a writer.

To ensure accuracy of both content and quotes, much research went into the development of this book. All those I interviewed took the time to review the text for accuracy; I thank them for their invaluable expertise and time. Sausalito Public Library reference librarian Keith Anderson, M.A., tracked down many invaluable sources and resources for me. I thank him especially and the other reference librarians who answered my questions and directed me to relevant resources.

From inception to completion, my agent Patti Breitman shared her expertise. I also appreciate the editorial support of Mary Jane Ryan, editor and publisher of Conari Press. Her insights nurtured the creative process and helped to sculpt the manuscript into a book.

Beyond words and expressions of thankfulness is the gratitude I feel for my husband, Larry Scherwitz, Ph.D. His grace-filled sensibilities, encouragement, and patience, our intellectual discussions, his many hours of creative support, early morning editing sessions, his "putting into practice" the concepts in this book and sharing his own personal vision quest, made this book possible.

To all those I have mentioned, please know that I am honored to have had the opportunity to talk with and learn from you. You so eloquently expressed your thoughts about the ancient human longing to find meaning in food and drink. Because of you, I learned much about the divine gift—and mystery—that is food. And because of you, the stream of deep human wisdom continues to flow.

notes

one: Spirituality: The Missing Ingredient in Food

1. Jean Anthelme Brillat-Savarin, "On the Pleasures of the Table," *The Physiology of Taste* (New York: Alfred A. Knopf, 1949), 183.

2. Huston Smith, *The Illustrated World's Religions: A Guide to Our Wisdom Traditions* (San Francisco: Harper San Francisco, 1994), 246.

3. D. Ornish, L. Scherwitz, R. Doody, and D. Kesten, et al., "Effects of Stress Management Training and Dietary Changes in Treating Ischemic Heart Disease," *Journal of the American Medical Association* 247 (1983): 54–59.

4. Deborah Kesten and Larry Scherwitz, et al., "Are Comprehensive Lifestyle Changes Possible in (European) Heart Patients?" *Progression and Regression of Atherosclerosis,* Koenig, ed., (Austria: Blackwell Wissenschaft, 1995).

5. Phone interview with Chevron publicist Bonnie Chaikind, February 13, 1996.

two: Judaism: Divine Dietary Tradition

1. Leon R. Kass, M.D., *The Hungry Soul: Eating and the Perfecting of Our Nature* (New York: The Free Press, 1994), 198.

2. Molly Cone, *Stories of Jewish Symbols* (New York: Bloch Publishing Company, 1963), 16–17.

3. Molly Cone, *The Jewish Sabbath* (New York: Thomas Y. Crowell Company, 1966).

4. Kass, *The Hungry Soul,* 196.

5. Richard Cavendish, ed., *Man, Myth and Magic: The Illustrated Encyclopedia of Mythology, Religion and the Unknown* (N. Bellmore, NY: Marshall Cavendish Corp., 1987), 12:97.

6. Personal conversation with Rabbi Harold Schulweis at Temple Valley Beth Shalom, Encino, California. Rabbi Schulweis is the

author of *For Those Who Can't Believe* (HarperCollins) and "Thou Shalt Eat Vegetables" in *Rabbis and Vegetarianism: An Evolving Tradition* (Marblehead, MA: Michah Publications, Inc., 1995).

7. Cavendish, *Man, Myth and Magic*, 1:388.

8. Ibid., 1:1435. Emphasis added.

9. Mary Douglas, *Purity and Danger: An Analysis of the Concepts of Pollution and Taboo* (London: Routledge, 1966), 57.

10. Rabbi Harold Schulweis, "Then the Holy One Came and Slaughtered the Angel of Death: Vegetarianism and Keeping Kosher," an edited version of which appears in *Rabbis and Vegetarianism*, 4.

11. Roberta Kalechofsky, ed., "Ethical Vegetarianism: The Perspective of a Reform Jew," *Rabbis and Vegetarianism: An Evolving Tradition* (Marblehead, MA: Micah Publications, Inc., 1995), 64.

12. Ibid., 65.

13. Max Friedman, "Food of the Gods," *Vegetarian Times*, August 1994, 61.

14. Schulweis, "Then the Holy One Came and Slaughtered the Angel of Death," 4.

15. Douglas, *Purity and Danger*, 29.

16. Kass, *The Hungry Soul*, 215.

17. Richard Schwartz, *Judaism and Vegetarianism* (Marblehead, MA: Micah Publications, Inc., 1988), 2.

18. *Encyclopedia Judaica* (Jerusalem, Israel: Keter Publishing House, Ltd., 1971), vol. 6.

19. Cavendish, *Man, Myth and Magic*, vol. 8.

20. Ibid.

21. Kalechofsky, "Ethical Vegetarianism," 83–84.

22. Douglas, *Purity and Danger*, 57.

23. Kass, *The Hungry Soul*, 216–224.

24. Phone interview with Richard Schwartz, Ph.D. Dr. Schwartz is a professor of mathematics at the College of Staten Island, Staten Island, New York. He is the author of *Judaism and Vegetarianism* (cited above), *Judaism and Global Survival* (New York: Atara Press, 1987), and *Mathematics and Global Survival* (Needham Heights, MA: Simon and Schuster, 1993).

25. Henri Daniel-Rops, *Daily Life in the Time of Jesus* (New York: Hawthorn Books, 1992), 228–229.

three: Christianity: The Sacred Supper

1. Personal conversation with Father Robert Bryant at the Episcopal Church of Our Savior, Mill Valley, California.

2. Alton H. McEachern, *Here at Thy Table, Lord: Enriching the Observance of the Lord's Supper* (Nashville, TN: Broadman Press, 1977), 95.

3. Kevin Orlin Johnson, Ph.D., *Why Do Catholics Do That: A Guide to the Teachings and Practices of the Catholic Church* (New York: Ballantine Books, 1994), 67.

4. Monika K. Hellwig, *The Eucharist and the Hunger of the World* (New York: Paulist Press, 1976), 22.

5. Phone interview with architect Arthur Manetta, Jr. from his home in Laguna Beach, California.

6. Father Robert Bryant, personal conversation.

7. Hughes Oliphant Old, "Rescuing Spirituality From the Cloister," *Christianity Today* 38, no. 7 (June 20, 1994): 27–29.

8. Mircea Eliade, ed., *The Encyclopedia of Religion* (New York: Macmillan Publishing Co., 1987), 5:185.

9. Cavendish, *Man, Myth and Magic,* 2:1668.

10. Ibid.

11. Arts and Entertainment, "The Last Supper," *Mysteries of the Bible,* aired November 21, 1996.

12. Personal interview with Clayton Harrop, Ph.D., former academic dean and vice president of academic affairs, professor of New Testament, at his office at Golden Gate Baptist Theological Seminary, Mill Valley, California. Dr. Harrop is the author of *History of the New Testament in Plain Language* (Waco, TX: Word Books, 1984) and other publications.

13. Arts and Entertainment, "The Last Supper."

14. George Galavaris, *Bread and the Liturgy: The Symbolism of Early Christian and Byzantine Bread Stamps* (Madison, WI: The University of Wisconsin Press, 1970), 4.

15. Hans Biedermann, *Dictionary of Symbolism: Cultural Icons and the Meanings Behind Them* (New York: Facts on File, Inc., 1992), 383.

16. Gertrude Jobes, *Dictionary of Mythology, Folklore and Symbolism, Part I* (New York: The Scarecrow Press, 1962), 244.

17. Eliade, *The Encyclopedia of Religion*, 8:490–491.

18. Ibid.

19. Ibid.

20. Jobes, *Dictionary of Mythology, Folklore and Symbolism*, 244.

21. Biedermann, *Dictionary of Symbolism*, 48.

22. Ibid., 49.

23. Galavaris, *Bread and the Liturgy*, 4.

24. Arts and Entertainment, "The Last Supper."

25. David Fontana, *The Secret Language of Symbols: A Visual Key to Symbols and Their Meanings* (London: Duncan Baird Publishers, 1993), 106.

26. Jobes, *Dictionary of Mythology, Folklore and Symbolism*, 1684.

27. J. C. Kooper, *An Illustrated Encyclopedia of Traditional Symbols* (London: Thames and Hudson, 1978), 193.

28. Cavendish, *Man, Myth and Magic*, 16:2257.

29. David S. Toolan, "At Home in the Cosmos: The Poetics of Matter-Energy," *America* 174, no. 6 (February 24, 1996), 8–14.

30. Personal interview with Jean Molesky-Poz at her office at the Department of Ethnic Studies, University of California, Berkeley.

31. Johnson, *Why Do Catholics Do That*, 68.

32. Phone interview with Jerry Scherwitz from his home in Sweetwater, Texas.

33. Caroline Walker Bynum, *Holy Feast and Holy Fast: The Religious Significance of Food to Medieval Women* (Berkeley, CA: University of California Press, 1987), 257.

34. Thomas Moore, *The Re-Enchantment of Everyday Life* (New York: HarperCollins Publishers, Inc., 1996), 62.

four: African Roots, American Soul Food

1. Evan Jones, *American Food: The Gastronomic Story* (New York: E. P. Dutton & Co., Inc., 1975), 83.

2. Josephine A. Beoku-Betts, "We Got Our Way of Cooking Things: Women, Food and Preservation of Cultural Identity...," *Gender and Society* 9, no. 5 (October 1995), 552.

3. Sheila Ferguson, *Soul Food: Classic Cuisine From the South* (New York: Grove Press, 1989), viii.

4. Jones, *American Food*, 86.

5. Beoku-Betts, "We Got Our Way of Cooking Things," 552.

6. Ibid., 547.

7. Jones, *American Food*, 89.

8. Margery S. Berube and staff, *The American Heritage Dictionary* (New York: Dell Publishing Co., Inc., 1983), 645.

9. Jones, *American Food*, 93.

five: India: Yogic Nutrition

1. Sanskrit prayer recited to me by former Swami Nischala Joy Devi, during a personal interview at her home in Fairfax, California.

2. Ray Barry, ed., *The Spiritual Athlete: A Primer for Inner Life* (Olema, CA: Joshua Press, 1992), 19.

3. Devi, personal interview.

4. O. M. Aivanhov, "Yoga Way of Eating," *Living Yoga: A Comprehensive Guide for Daily Life,* Georg Feuerstein and Stephan Bodian, eds., (New York: J. P. Tarcher/Perigee, 1993), 103–104.

5. Personal interview with cardiologist Dr. K. L. Chopra at the "First International Conference on Lifestyle and Health," New Delhi, India, January 1994.

6. Personal interview with spiritual teacher Swami Dharmananda at the Adhyathma Sadhana Kendra Yoga Center, New Delhi, India, January 1994.

7. Aivanhov, "Yoga Way of Eating," 98.

8. Ibid., "Yoga Way of Eating," 104.

9. Vivian Worthington, *A History of Yoga* (London: Arkana, 1989), 181.

10. Swami Satchidananda, "Healthful Hints on Eating Habits and Diet," educational handout distributed by the Integral Yoga Institute, Satchidananda Ashram (Buckingman, VA: Yogaville, Inc.).

six: Islam: Devout Dining

1. Ahmad H. Sakr, Ph.D., *Dietary Regulations and Food Habits of Muslims* (New York: Muslim World League, Makkah Mukarramah, 1976), 6.

2. Islamic Affairs Department, "Understanding Islam and the Muslims," (Washington, DC: Embassy of Saudi Arabia, n.d.).

3. Ibid.

4. Florence Mary Fitch, *Allah: The God of Islam* (New York: Lothrop, Lee & Shepard Co., Inc., 1950), 47.

5. Eliade, *The Encyclopedia of Religion,* 4:405.

6. Personal interview with Ameena Jandali at her home in El Cerrito, California.

7. Audiocassette-recorded information from Ahmad Sakr, Ph.D., formerly a professor and chairman of the Department of Chemistry and Nutrition at the National College of Chiropractic in Lombard, Illinois, and founder of the Foundation For Islamic Knowledge in Walnut, California. Dr. Sakr has written many books, pamphlets, and brochures about Islamic practices.

8. Personal interview with Hamid Algar, Ph.D., professor of Islamic Studies, at his office at the University of California, Berkeley.

9. Cavendish, *Man, Myth and Magic*, 1:102.

10. John F. Wrynn, "Ramadan is Generous," *America* 172, no. 17, 22.

11. Imad-Ad-Dean Ahmad and Syed Khalid Shaukat, "Muslim Moon-Sightings," *Mercury* (May-June, 1995).

12. Sakr, *Dietary Regulations and Food Habits of Muslims*, 6.

13. M. Cherif Bassiouni, *Introduction to Islam* (New York: Rand McNally, 1988), 39.

14. Ibid.

15. Raymond Lifchez, ed., *The Dervish Lodge: Architecture, Art, and Sufism in Ottoman Turkey* (Berkeley and Los Angeles: University of California Press, Ltd., 1992), 302.

16. Lifchez, *The Dervish Lodge*, 302.

17. Sakr, *Dietary Regulations and Food Habits of Muslims*, 6.

18. Sakr, audiocassette-recorded information.

seven: Buddhism: Mindful Meals

1. Abbot John Daido Loori, *Master Dogen's Metaphysics of Eating* (Mt. Tremper, NY: Dharma Communications, 1994), audiocassette.

2. Zen Mountain Monastery, *Oryoki Formal Monastery Meal: Master Dogen's Instructions for a Miraculous Occasion* (Mt. Tremper, NY: Dharma Communications, 1994), videocassette.

3. Ibid., "Chant Sheet" supplement. Begin chanting with hands

pressed together in a traditional *gassho* mudra, which is a mudra of identity, with both hands (symbolically) becoming one entity. Position hands several inches in front of face.

4. After the word "food," wrap the right hand around the left fist at the waist, resting both hands in the lap; at the same time, bow (while seated) from the waist.

5. After this first sentence, straighten up and change the *shushu* mudra into the cosmic mudra: fingertips and palms resting together and touching, leaving a slight "oval" between palms; position hands at waist level, resting in the lap.

6. After this fifth sentence, place hands in *gassho* and bow. Then take a mere pinch (perhaps ⅛ teaspoon) of food from the Buddha bowl, touch the food to your forehead, then place the food on the tip of a utensil (spatula handle) as an offering. Then return hands to the traditional prayer mudra.

7. Bow slightly, with hands held in the prayer mudra.

8. Bow slightly, then raise the Buddha bowl until it is just above eye level. Retaining this position, complete the remainder of the chant.

9. At end of the chant, bow; begin eating with Buddha bowl held in hands, taking the first morsel of food from the Buddha bowl.

10. This part of the *Oryoki* ritual is performed only at the lunch meal, accompanied by this chanted phrase: *All those of the spiritual worlds, now I give you this offering. This food will pervade everywhere.*

11. "Chant Sheet" supplement.

12. Ibid.

13. Zen Mountain Monastery, *Oryoki Formal Monastery Meal,* video-cassette.

14. Ibid.

15. Ibid.

16. Personal interview with Yvonne Rand at her home and meditation center in West Marin, California. Rand is a Zen Buddhist priest and meditation teacher who is active in working for

Tibetan causes. She and her husband Bill Sterling are cofounders of the Society for the Preservation of Gyoto Sacred Arts.

17. Eliade, *The Encyclopedia of Religion,* vol. 5.

18. Ibid., vol. 4.

19. Ibid., vol. 5.

20. Joseph F. Rock, "Life Among the Lamas of Choni," *National Geographic* (Washington, DC: National Geographic Society, 1928), 606.

21. Personal interview with Lama Kunga Rinpoche, Tibetan high lama, founder and teacher, at the Tibetan Buddhist Meditation Center (Ewam Choden), Kensington, California. Its mission is to provide an opportunity for practitioners to study Tibetan religion and culture. He is the author of *Drinking From the Mountain Stream* and *Miraculous Journey.* Kunga Rinpoche's father, Tibetan nobleman Tsipon Shuguba, is the author of *In the Presence of My Enemies,* an autobiography about his nineteen-year imprisonment after the Chinese invasion of Tibet and Tibetan military resistance.

22. Lama Thubten Yeshe, *Introduction to Tantra: A Vision of Totality* (Boston: Wisdom Publications, 1987), 163.

23. Rock, "Life Among the Lamas of Choni," 606.

24. Kunga Rinpoche, personal interview.

25. Linda Johnsen, "Rediscovering Tantra," *Yoga Journal* (January/February 1996), 30.

26. Personal interview with Carol Corradi, Tibetan nun and director of Tse Chen Ling Center, San Francisco, California, whose mission is to provide an opportunity for people to receive Buddhist teachings.

27. Thubten Yeshe, *Introduction to Tantra,* 160.

28. Ibid.

29. Ibid, 163.

30. Loori, *Master Dogen's Metaphysics of Cooking,* audiocassette.

31. Thich Nhat Hanh, *Peace is Every Step: The Path of Mindfulness in Everyday Life* (New York: Bantam Books, 1992), 24.

eight: China and Japan: Food Folklore, Tea Treasure

1. Carol Stepanchuk and Charles Wong, *Mooncakes and Hungry Ghosts: Festivals of China* (San Francisco: China Books & Periodicals, Inc., 1991), 131.

2. Eelco Hesse, *Tea: The Eyelids of Bodhidharma* (Great Britain: Prism Press, 1982), 26.

3. John Blofeld, *The Chinese Art of Tea* (Boston: Shambhala Publications, Inc., 1985).

4. Stepanchuk and Wong, *Mooncakes and Hungry Ghosts*, 4.

5. Ibid.

6. Ibid., 6.

7. Alain Y. Dessaint, "The Chinese Way of Eating," *Natural History* (August-September 1977), 102.

8. Personal interview with Suk Wah Bernstein, a writer and yoga practitioner, in Oakland, California.

9. David Lee Hoffman, "Leaf & Water...an adventure in simplicity," (Lagunitas, CA: Silk Road Teas), brochure.

10. Matthew Stafford, "Taking Tea," *Pacific Sun*, September 4–10, 1996.

11. Sen Soshitsu XV, *The Urasenke Tradition of Tea* (Kyoto, Japan: Urasenke Foundation, 1983), 4.

12. Kakuzo Okakura, *The Book of Tea* (Boston and London: Shambhala, 1993), 81.

13. Ibid., 1.

14. Ibid., 36.

15. Ibid., 53.

16. Ibid., 28.

17. Eliade, *The Encyclopedia of Religion*, 2:120.

18. Personal interview with Christy A. Bartlett at the Urasenke Foundation, San Francisco, California. To delve further into both the spiritual and secular teachings of the art of the tea, I visited her and Scott McDougal, a student and teacher of the Way of Tea, at the Urasenke Foundation, established by Bartlett in 1981 as a representative of Sen Soshitsu XV, fifteenth-generation Grand Tea Master of the Urasenke Tradition of Chanoyu in Kyoto, Japan.

19. Urasenke Foundation, "The Urasenke Tradition of Chado," (Kyoto, Japan: Urasenke Foundation, 1995).

20. Hesse, *Tea: The Eyelids of Bodhidharma*, 27.

21. Okakura, *The Book of Tea*, 3.

22. Public Affairs Television, transcript from "Bill Moyers: The Wisdom of Faith with Huston Smith, Part 2: Confucianism," aired April 2, 1996.

23. Lois Maclean, "Midnight Supper," *Pacific Sun*, March 15–21, 1995.

nine: Native American: The Vision Quest Fast

1. Eliade, "Quests," The *Encyclopedia of Religion*, 12:147.

2. Joseph Epes Brown, *Animals of the Soul: Sacred Animals of the Oglala Sioux* (Rockport, MA: Element, Inc., 1992), 52.

3. Ibid., 54.

4. Phone interview with Native American Katie Martin from her home in Oregon. She and her husband, David, a spiritual healer, also have a home in Minneapolis, Minnesota.

5. Eliade, *The Encyclopedia of Religion*, 5:287.

6. Ibid., 287–288.

ten: Hinduism: The Wedding Feast

1. M. F. K. Fisher, "Here Let Us Feast: A Book of Banquets," *Dubious Honors* (San Francisco: North Point Press, 1988), 156.

2. Eliade, *The Encyclopedia of Religion*, 4:60.

3. Cavendish, *Man, Myth and Magic*, vol. 12.

4. Ibid.

5. Eliade, *The Encyclopedia of Religion*, 9:33.

6. The description of the wedding of Nutan Sharma and Arthur Brownstein is derived from a personal interview I conducted with Nutan in my home, and from the videocassette of their wedding ceremony that she so kindly loaned me for clarification and edification.

7. Eliade, *The Encyclopedia of Religion*, 9:408.

8. During a phone interview, information about the symbolism that surrounds the Hindu marital fire and food was given to me by Pandit Hari Shankar Dabral of the Himalayan Institute of Yoga Science and Philosophy, Glen View, Illinois.

9. Fisher, "Here Let Us Feast: A Book of Banquets," 157.

10. Eliade, *The Encyclopedia of Religion*, 9:33.

11. Burt Wolf, *Gatherings and Celebrations* (New York: Doubleday, 1996), p. x.

12. Daniel-Rops, *Daily Life in the Time of Jesus*.

eleven: Enlightened Eating

1. Barbara McNeill, ed., *Noetic Sciences Review* (Winter 1996), 4.

2. Ibid., 5.

3. Michelle Stacey, *Consumed: Why Americans Love, Hate, and Fear Food* (New York: Touchstone, 1994).

4. Ibid.

twelve: Eating Disorders: The Starving Spirit

1. R. S. Jones, "The Very, Very Thin Man," *Mademoiselle,* February 1994, 112.

2. Personal interview with psychologist Susan Boulware, Ph.D., at her office in Sausalito, California.

3. Joan Jacobs Brumberg, *Fasting Girls: The History of Anorexia Nervosa* (Cambridge, MA: Harvard University Press, 1988), 12.

4. Jean Seligman, "The Pressure to Lose," *Newsweek* May 2, 1994, 60.

5. Jean Callahan, "Update on Eating Disorders," *Cosmopolitan* May 1996, 232.

6. Ibid., 233.

7. Laura Shapiro, "A Food Lover's Guide to Fat," *Newsweek* December 1994.

8. Carolyn O'Neil, correspondent, "Food to Die For," *CNN Presents*, aired November 20, 1994.

9. Food Survey Research Group, United States Department of Agriculture, "Continuing Survey of Food Intakes by Individuals 1994," (Riverdale, MD: Agricultural Research Service).

10. "Body/Mind" column, *Self* December 1995, 63.

11. National Association of Anorexia & Associated Disorders, "ANAD: Facts About Eating Disorders," "Media Page," fact sheets dated April 25, 1996 (Highland Park, IL: ANAD).

12. Brumberg, *Fasting Girls*, 165.

13. David Riesman, *The Lonely Crowd* (New Haven, CT: University Press, 1950).

14. Phone interview with psychologist Michael Mayer, Ph.D., from his home in Orinda, California.

15. Alexander Lowen, M.D., *Narcissism: Denial of the True Self* (New York: Macmillan Publishing Co., 1985), 26.

16. H. Kirschenbaum and V. L. Henderson, eds., *The Carl Rogers Reader* (Boston: Houghton Mifflin Co., 1989), 155.

17. Ibid., 156.

18. Journal Graphics, Inc., "Princess Diana: The Interview," *ABC News: Turning Point*, aired November 24, 1995. Transcript #151 (American Broadcasting Companies, 1995), 4.

19. Alice Miller, *The Drama of the Gifted Child* (New York: Basic Books, Inc., 1981).

20. Radio interview with Melody Marks, M.S.W., on "The Michael Krasny Show" (San Francisco), ABC-KGO Newstalk Radio, broadcast December 20, 1990.

21. Boulware, personal interview.

22. Journal Graphics, Inc., "The Hunger Inside," *ABC News: 20/20*, aired December 2, 1994. Transcript #1448 (American Broadcasting Companies, Inc., 1994), 8.

23. Callahan, "Update on Eating Disorders," 232.

24. Burrell's Transcripts, "Male Eating Disorders," *Oprah: The Oprah Winfrey Show*, aired January 17, 1996 (Harpo Productions, Inc., 1996), 13–14.

25. Journal Graphics, Inc., "The Hunger Inside," 4.

26. Ibid., 5–10.

27. Jacquelyn Small, M.S.S.W., *Transformers: The Therapists of the Future* (Marina del Rey, CA: DeVorss & Co., 1982), 18.

28. Ibid., 17.

29. Ibid., 221.

30. Jo Ind, *Fat is a Spiritual Issue: My Journey* (New York: Mowbray, 1993), 95.

31. Ibid., 94–95.

32. Ibid.

33. Ibid., 96

34. Leonard Laskow, M.D., *Healing with Love* (San Francisco: HarperCollins, 1992), 3–4.

35. Victoria Moran, *The Love-Powered Diet: A Revolutionary Approach to*

Healthy Eating and Recovery From Food Addiction (San Rafael, CA: New World Library, 1992), 19–20. Reissued in 1997 by Daybreak Books (Rodale) under the title *Love Yourself Thin: How to Stop Eating When You Don't Want to Eat, Eat Healthy When You Do, and Love Your Body All the Time.*

36. Ibid., 21.

37. Ibid., 25–26.

38. Paul Wilner, "Editor's Note," *San Francisco Examiner Magazine* (August 6, 1995). From the poem "Bread and Roses" (1912) by James Oppenheim.

thirteen: The Food-Mood Connection

1. Carrie Angus, M.D., "Food for the Wise," *Yoga International* March/April, 1996, 22.

2. Judith J. Wurtman, *Managing Your Mind and Mood Through Food* (New York: Rawson Associates, 1986), 7.

3. Ibid.

4. Phone interview with nutritionist and food-mood specialist Catherine Christie, Ph.D., R.D., from her office in Jacksonville, Florida.

5. Research cited in Elizabeth Somer, M.A., R.D., "Irrestible Urges," *Shape* January 1994, 34–35.

6. Debra Waterhouse, M.P.H., R.D., *Why Women Need Chocolate: Eat What You Crave to Look and Feel Great* (New York: Hyperion, 1995).

7. Jean Carper, *Food — Your Miracle Medicine* (New York: HarperCollins, 1993), 274.

8. Elizabeth Somer, *Food and Mood: The Complete Guide to Feeling Well and Eating Your Best* (New York: Holt, 1994).

9. Elizabeth Somer, "The Anti-Anxiety Diet," *Self* January 1995, 117.

10. Carper, *Food — Your Miracle Medicine*, 274.

11. Ibid.

12. Ibid.

13. Ibid.

14. Wurtman, *Managing Your Mind and Mood Through Food*, 7.

fourteen: Spiritually Imbued Food

1. Deepak Chopra, "Body, Mind and Soul," KQED-TV presentation, aired March 7, 1995. (San Francisco: Public Broadcasting Station).

2. Phone interview with Larry Dossey, M.D. An internist, Dr. Dossey has written about the power of prayer, consciousness, and spirituality and is a pioneer in an emerging field that studies the effects of prayer and consciousness on the healing process. He publishes *Alternative Therapies* and is the author of *Healing Words*, *Meaning and Medicine*, *Recovering the Soul*, *Beyond Illness*, and *Space, Time and Medicine*.

3. Personal interview with Marilyn Schlitz, Ph.D., director of research at the Institute of Noetic Sciences, Sausalito, California.

4. Jeffrey Mishlove, Ph.D., with Fred Alan Wolf, Ph.D., "Physics and Consciousness," based on the PBS production *Thinking Allowed* (Oakland, CA: Thinking Allowed Productions, 1988), videocassette. Emphasis added.

5. Phone interview with Rev. Dr. Karl Goodfellow from his home in Guttenberg, Iowa, regarding his statewide research project about the affects of prayer on farmers' harvest and farm safety. Rev. Dr. Goodfellow is the minister of the United Methodist Church in Guttenberg.

6. P. Tompkins and C. Bird, *The Secret Life of Plants* (New York, Harper & Row, 1972), 5.

7. Ibid, 6.

8. Ibid.

9. Leonard Laskow, M.D., *Healing with Love: A Breakthrough Mind/Body Medical Program for Healing Yourself and Others* (San Francisco, Harper San Francisco, 1992), 35–36.

10. P. Tompkins, and C. Bird, *The Secret Life of Plants*, 354.

11. Phone interview with Larry Dossey, M.D., from his home in Sante Fe, New Mexico.

12. Personal interview with Leonard Laskow, M.D., at his office in Mill Valley, California.

13. Personal interview with Ali Babajane at his Champs-Elysée Restaurant in Sausalito, California.

14. Personal interview with Irene Averell at my home in Sausalito, California.

15. Laskow, personal interview.

fifteen: Food Meditation: Creating Conscious Connection

1. O. M. Aivanhov, *The Yoga of Nutrition* (Frejus, France: Prosveta, 1982), 3

2. Burrell's Transcripts, "Resolutions That Matter," *Oprah: The Oprah Winfrey Show*, aired January 16, 1997 (Harpo Productions, Inc., 1997), 17.

3. Alan Watts, *Alan Watts Seminars: Theory and Practice of Meditation*, Sausalito Public Library, videotape #C427.

4. Personal interview with stress management specialist Jon Kabat-Zinn, Ph.D., in San Francisco, California.

5. Jon Kabat-Zinn, *Full Catastrophe Living* (New York: Delacorte Press, 1990), 440.

6. Cavendish, *Man, Myth and Magic*, 12:1677–1680.

7. Ibid.

8. Eliade, *The Encyclopedia of Religion*, 325.

9. Ibid.

10. Phone interview with psychologist Michael Mayer, Ph.D., from his home in Orinda, California.

11. To learn more about Yichuan, Dr. Mayer suggests *The Nature of Energy* by Fong Ha (Berkeley, CA: Summerhouse Publications, 1996).

12. Prince Charles, advertisement in *Style* July 1995, 54.

13. Sue Bender, *Everyday Sacred* (San Francisco: HarperCollins San Francisco, 1995).

14. Phone interview with Valerie Phipps, co-owner of Phipps Ranch, in Pescadero, California.

index